CLINICAL COACH

for

Effective Pain Management

Davis's

CLINICAL
COACH

Series

CLINICAL COACH

COACH

for

Effective Pain Management

Paul Arnstein, RN, PhD
Clinical Nurse Specialist for
Pain Relief
Massachusetts General Hospital
Boston, Massachusetts

F.A. Davis Company • Philadelphia

F. A. Davis Company
1915 Arch Street
Philadelphia, PA 19103
www.fadavis.com

Printed in China

Last digit indicates print number: 10 9 8 7 6 5 4 3 2 1

Publisher, Nursing: Joanne Patzek DaCunha, RN, MSN
Director of Content Development: Darlene D. Pedersen
Senior Developmental Editor: William Welsh
Project Editor: Tyler R. Baber
Cover Design: Carolyn O'Brien

As new scientific information becomes available through basic and clinical research, recommended treatments and drug therapies undergo changes. The author(s) and publisher have done everything possible to make this book accurate, up to date, and in accord with accepted standards at the time of publication. The author(s), editors, and publisher are not responsible for errors or omissions or for consequences from application of the book, and make no warranty, expressed or implied, in regard to the contents of the book. Any practice described in this book should be applied by the reader in accordance with professional standards of care used in regard to the unique circumstances that may apply in each situation. The reader is advised always to check product information (package inserts) for changes and new information regarding dose and contraindications before administering any drug. Caution is especially urged when using new or infrequently ordered drugs.

Library of Congress Cataloging-in-Publication Data

Arnstein, Paul, 1956-
    Clinical coach for effective pain management / Paul Arnstein.
        p. ; cm.
    Includes bibliographical references and index.
    ISBN-13: 978-0-8036-2175-6
    ISBN-10: 0-8036-2175-2
1. Pain—Nursing. 2. Pain. I. Title.
    [DNLM: 1. Pain—nursing. 2. Nursing Care—methods. 3. Pain—therapy.
WY 160.5 A767c 2010]
    RT87.P35A76 2010
    616'.0472—dc22

                                                                    2009044274

To my lovely wife, Honor, who is
always first in my book.

Reviewers

Paula Boley, EdD, MSN, RN
Professor and Graduate Coordinator
School of Nursing
Anderson University
Anderson, Indiana

Barbara A. Bonenberger, RN, BSN, MNEd, CNE
Instructor
University of Pittsburgh School of Nursing
Pittsburgh, Pennsylvania

Erla Champ-Gibson, BSN, MDiv, PhD student
Instructor of Nursing
Seattle Pacific University
Seattle, Washington

Carmela Theresa de Leon, BSN, RN, MAN
Faculty Member
PIMA Medical Institute
Active Medical Surgical RN, Orthopedics and Bariatrics
Banner Gateway Medical Center
Mesa, Arizona

Kristen Fenlason, MS, RN
Adult Health Nursing Instructor
Lake Superior College
Duluth, Minnesota

Priscilla Gage Gwyn, ARNP-BC, MSN, CNS, OCN®
Assistant Professor
Florida Hospital College of Health Sciences
Orlando, Florida

Juanita Landers, MSN, CRNP, CDE
Clinical Instructor
Auburn University Montgomery
Montgomery, Alabama

Kathleen A. LuPone, MS, CNRN, FNP-BC
Clinical Assistant Professor, Nurse Practitioner
in Adult Neurology
College of Nursing and Healthcare Innovation
Arizona State University
Barrows Neurological Institute in Neuroscience Critical Care
Gilbert Neurology in Private Practice
Phoenix, Arizona

Susan Madson, BSN, MSN
Professor of Nursing
Horry Georgetown Technical College
Conway, South Carolina

Lora McGuire RN, MS
Professor of Nursing
Joliet Junior College
Joliet, Illinois

Susan A. Moore, RN, PhD
Assistant Professor, Nursing
University of Memphis
Memphis, Tennessee

Margaret O'Brien King, PhD, RN-BC, AHN-BC, CNL
Professor, Nursing
College of Social Sciences, Health, and Education
Xavier University
Cincinnati, Ohio

Thomas L. Petricini, RN, MSN
Nursing Instructor
Sharon Regional Health System
Sharon, Pennsylvania

Mary Ellen Pike, RN, MSN, MA, PhD candidate
Assistant Professor
Bellarmine University
Louisville, Kentucky

Judith Stanley, RN, MS, DHSc
Assistant Professor of Nursing
D'Youville College
Buffalo, New York

Delores (Lori) Stephens, MN, RN, CLNC
Nursing Faculty
Skagit Valley College
Mount Vernon, Washington

Barbara Kim Stevens, MSN, RN, DNP
Assistant Professor of Nursing
University of Rio Grande–Holzer School of Nursing
Rio Grande, Ohio

Thelma Stich, PhD, RN
President & Owner
Student Nurse Coach LLC
Staten Island, New York

Christine M. Thomas, RN, MSN, DNSc
Associate Professor
West Chester University
West Chester, Pennsylvania

April Hazard Vallerand, PhD, RN, FAAN
Associate Professor
Wayne State University College of Nursing
Detroit, Michigan

Bruce Wilson, PhD, RN, CNS
Professor, Department of Nursing
University of Texas-Pan American
Edinburg, Texas

Diane Young, PhD, CNE, RN
Professor, Nursing Department
Allen College
Waterloo, Iowa

Table of Contents

1 The Nurse's Role in Pain Control

CHAPTER 1

The Nurse's Role in Pain Control

Getting Started

Improving pain management begins with the self-development and professional development of the individual nurse. Nurses must explore their own levels of knowledge and skills and their personal and cultural attitudes that will affect their ability to understand, assess, and manage pain. Attitudes or values about drug use or nondrug interventions might produce subtle yet important biases when interacting with patients experiencing pain. Reach out and network with colleagues who are committed to quality pain management. Be familiar with professional organizations, clinical guidelines, position papers, and other resources that focus on pain management. Additionally, being open-minded, committing to lifelong learning, seeking assistance when uncertainties arise, and becoming an effective member of the interdisciplinary team will enhance the nurse's ability to promote optimal pain control.

This book was developed to provide nurses with the tools needed to care for patients with pain. The nurse who masters the content of this reference will be able to:

- Identify barriers to pain control
- Describe the nurses' duty to manage pain
- Apply current theories and knowledge about pain to clinical scenarios
- Distinguish acute pain, chronic pain, and pain associated with life-limiting illnesses
- Assess the physical, emotional, social, and spiritual aspects of pain

- Safely administer prescribed analgesia using a variety of routes and monitor, record, and evaluate its effectiveness
- Use the nursing processes to assess, identify desired outcomes, plan, implement, and evaluate pain in a systematic manner
- Describe a variety of invasive and noninvasive treatments available in addition to medication to enhance physical and psychosocial comfort
- Differentiate addiction from aberrant drug behaviors, physical dependence, tolerance, and pseudoaddiction

The Problem of Pain

Pain is a universal experience; it is the reason why many seek health care [1] and it is very costly to society [2–5]. Pain commonly is thought of as a necessary part of birth, life, and death; however, effective pain treatments can be used throughout the life span. At its best, pain is a vital physiological warning system, alerting the person that urgent attention is needed to prevent injury or death. At its worst, it is an incurable disease. The person afflicted with persistent pain often becomes an unwilling burden on others and may fight a losing battle to have others believe and relieve the pain.

Despite scientific and professional advances in pain relief, patients still experience needless pain and suffering. Unrelieved pain is harmful: it interferes with healing, immunity, functioning, [6–8] and puts patients at risk for developing complications.

Barriers to Effective Treatment of Pain

Pain often is untreated or undertreated, despite the availability of effective treatments. Although some pain is refractory to treatment, the majority of pain-control failures result from:
- Professional barriers—personal biases and inadequate knowledge or skills
- Patient barriers—fears (medication dangers), incorrect assumptions, poor communication, and passivity
- System barriers—restrictive laws, policies, and limited access to treatment

Common to all these barriers are concerns related to:
- Inadequate pain assessment
- Mistaken beliefs about pain and available treatments (see Box 1–1 for definitions of pain)
- Exaggerated fears associated with use of opioids*

Box 1–1 Definitions of Pain

For scientific and clinical purposes, the International Association for the Study of Pain (IASP) defines pain as "an unpleasant sensory and emotional experience associated with actual or potential tissue damage, or described in terms of such damage."[†]

The most commonly cited definition in clinical nursing, which was first given more than 40 years ago by Margo McCaffery is: "Pain is whatever the experiencing person says it is, existing whenever he (the experiencing person) says it does."[††]

IASP and McCaffery later clarify that the inability to communicate verbally does not negate the possibility that pain is being experienced and appropriate pain-relieving treatment is needed.

[†]Merskey H., Bogduk N. (Eds.). (1994). *Classification of chronic pain and definitions of pain terms* (2nd ed., p. 213). Seattle: IASP Press.
[††]McCaffery M., Pasero C. (1999). *Pain clinical manual* (2nd ed., p. 17). St. Louis, Mosby.

Personal and Social Beliefs that Prevent Effective Treatment

To provide competent and ethically sound pain treatment, nurses need to reflect on how their own personal and professional experiences, values, beliefs, and cultures may serve as potential learned barriers to quality pain control [9]. The following feelings, biases, and attitudes on the part of a nurse can adversely affect pain treatment:

- Considering stoicism more appropriate than unrestrained emotional expression
- Preferring problem-focused coping styles over emotion-focused coping
- Believing only verifiable pain is real and other types of pain are "all in the head"
- Expecting a certain degree of pain based on a specific diagnosis or procedure
- Believing that a patient is drug seeking, solely on the basis of
  - Pain medication requests or
  - Lifestyle, diagnosis, or demographic factors
- Believing that the nurse is a better judge of the intensity of pain than the patient
- Believing that pain is punishment for sins or wrongdoing

*The term *opioid* is preferred over *narcotic* because the latter is a legal designation that encompasses several drug classes and has a social stigma attached to it.

By recognizing these potential barriers to optimal pain treatment, nurses can better identify situations where therapeutic failure may occur and act accordingly.

Nursing Role and Responsibility

Pain relief is an essential part of nursing practice. Every nurse, regardless of his or her role, specialty, or setting, has the responsibility to [10]:

- Protect patients from injury and the development or advancement of disease
- Alleviate suffering
- Advocate for the care needed by individuals, families, communities, and populations
- Work collaboratively with patients, families, and other health-care providers
- Practice nursing independently, using the nursing process to guide care

To carry out these responsibilities, the nurse must be knowledgeable and skilled in the assessment and management of pain. This involves the following skills:

- Developing and maintaining a working knowledge of
  - Pain assessment
  - Pharmacological and nondrug interventions
  - Equipment and resources used to promote safe, effective relief
- Developing skills in education, counseling, and patient advocacy
  - Maintaining a patient-centered focus, a helpful attitude, and a trusting therapeutic relationship
  - Respecting the patient's autonomy
  - Treating patients in a fair nonjudgmental manner
  - Upholding patients' rights to have their pain assessed and managed
  - Believing patients' reports about their perceived feelings and needs

Optimal pain management requires nurses to know the patient, including physical aspects of medical conditions and treatment and psychosocial

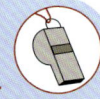

COACH CONSULT

Know Your Patient. The importance of knowing the patient is highlighted by the following story. Bill was admitted for incision and drainage of a cyst. After surgery, he writhed and cried, screaming in apparent pain. The nurses rapidly titrated his morphine to the point where he had to be placed on a ventilator because of his obesity and behavior suggestive of severe pain. When he was taken off the ventilator 2 months later, they learned that he was crying because his girlfriend broke up with him just before surgery.

and spiritual aspects related to pain and its effects. Each dimension can amplify or diminish the intensity of perceived pain. For example, when local anesthetics are not used, patients having vascular access devices inserted will invariably experience some discomfort. The identical procedure will elicit less pain if a caring nurse takes time to comfort the patient, explain the procedure, allay the patient's fears, and listen to his or her concerns than it would if the nurse did not attend to these psychosocial details.

Responsibility to Identify and Assess Pain

Because nurses are often the health professionals with the most frequent patient contact, they are in the best position to identify patients in pain. One should not assume a pain-free state when observing a child playing a video game, a young woman sitting quietly, or an old man lying still with his eyes closed. The nurse should screen each patient for pain with a simple question, such as, "Are you having any discomfort?" When discomfort is present, a more in-depth assessment is conducted. There are a variety of validated pain assessment tools and techniques useful for different patient populations detailed in the assessment chapter. An effective pain assessment tool is:

- Easy to use
- Sensitive enough to detect changes over time and responses to interventions
- Yields clinically meaningful data (i.e., evidence-based and is easy for patients to use).

A multidimensional pain assessment should yield more than just a number on a pain scale. It also should help the nurse to:

- Determine the underlying cause or mechanism of pain
- Monitor the patient's overall condition and progress (including emergence of complications)
- Explore psychosocial factors related to pain
- Identify risks/strategies by determining prior responses to pain and its treatment
- Identify patient barriers to pain relief (e.g., refusal to report pain or to use drugs)

Responsibility to Establish a Nursing Diagnosis and Treatment Plan

Pain is the most common nursing diagnosis used in clinical practice. When establishing a nursing diagnosis of pain, the nurse also must determine:

- Types of pain (acute, chronic, and mixed types)
- Underlying causes
- How pain is manifested (pain behaviors)

Based on these details, the nurse establishes a prioritized treatment plan designed to meet the patient's needs. Planning is based on goals for comfort and functioning developed mutually with the patient. This plan is further aligned with the treatment plan established collaboratively with the physician and interdisciplinary team. The nurse's role in pain relief is an active one.

Before implementing medical orders, the nurse should express any concerns to the prescriber. These may include:

- Mismatch between treatment and actual/anticipated pain (e.g., aspirin for postoperative pain)
- Drug contraindicated for the patient (e.g., agonist-antagonist type of analgesic for an opioid-tolerant patient)
- Drug or doses likely to be ineffective or to have a high side effect burden
- Failure to order baseline daily opioids for patients on long-term opioid therapy

If the prescriber is unwilling to accommodate justified requests by the nurse on behalf of the patient's plan of care, the nurse can request a consultation with an appropriate specialist or secure help based on the organization's resources and chain of command.

Responsibility to Intervene to Alleviate or Manage Pain

Nurses must intervene to relieve pain based on the assessment data and priorities established in the treatment plan. This typically involves a multimodal approach that includes pharmacological and nondrug therapies. Opioid analgesics are the cornerstone of treatment for moderate and severe pain. Nonopioid analgesics, such as acetaminophen, aspirin, and other NSAIDs are useful for mild to moderate pain and are used for severe pain to enhance opioid potency.

 NURSE-TO-NURSE TIP

The Ask. The ability to give information succinctly over the phone to get treatment adjustments is an important skill. Gather, summarize, and prioritize information, and practice "the ask." First identify yourself, the patient, the situation, and the patient's responses. For example, "I am nurse Ed Voquet caring for Ms. Handalin on the day after surgery. She received the maximum 2 tablets of Tylenol #3 every 4 hours as ordered without side effects, but is refusing to move because of unrelieved severe pain." Then ask, "Can we try a different medication to better reduce the pain, improve her breathing, ambulation, and participation in therapy?"

Pain medications often are ordered using range orders or on a prn basis. Nursing judgment determines what, when, and how much analgesic should be administered. Suggestions for optimizing the effectiveness of ordered prn and range-order medications include:

- Consider overall patient condition (i.e., anticipate safety and efficacy needs)
- Administer the first dose of analgesic
  - Start opioid-naïve patients at the lower end of the dose range
  - Start opioid-tolerant patients (daily opioids > 1 week) just above their usual dose
- Evaluate the safety (sedation, respirations) and efficacy of the dose within 1 hour, preferably at peak of effectiveness:
  - 15 minutes after IV administration
  - 30 to 60 minutes after intramuscular (IM) administration
  - 60 minutes after oral administration
- Barring sedation or respiratory depression, if pain is not satisfactorily relieved (cut to half of the pre-dose intensity level)
  - Administer an additional dose if permitted and within the limits of the order,
  - With a fixed-dose prn order, repeat the dose as soon as due, and administer another analgesic (e.g., acetaminophen) if ordered
- Offer subsequent prn doses when due; administer all prn doses, unless refused
- Administer or offer subsequent range-order doses on schedule. Base dosage on:
  - Prior response to analgesics (i.e., pain relief, side effects, and functioning)
  - Anticipated illness trajectory and duration of pain
  - Drug characteristics (i.e., onset, peak, duration of action)

COACH CONSULT

Use of a treatment protocol or set of standard orders decreases the use of potentially dangerous analgesics and encourages the use of antiemetics and laxatives to reduce the side effects of opioids. For example, a protocol might include acetaminophen, NSAIDs, or codeine for mild pain, hydrocodone, or oxycodone-containing medications for moderate pain, and morphine or hydromorphone for severe pain [11].

COACH CONSULT

Timing of reassessment after administering analgesic medications is particularly important in establishing the safety and efficacy of the drug. The best time to assess a drug's analgesic, sedative, and respiratory depressant effects is at the peak of effectiveness, which varies by drug and route. Exceptions to this rule are spinal morphine and methadone administered by any route—with these drugs, respiratory depression may occur hours after the analgesic effect has worn off.

When to Request a Change in Analgesia Regimen

If a drug is administered on schedule (e.g., every 4 hours) for 3 doses in the highest amounts ordered, without providing relief, the nurse should request an adjustment to the analgesic regimen. Nurses should concurrently use other available medications and nondrug pain relief measures to make the patient as comfortable as possible when pain persists. By the end of the 3rd dose, most short-acting drugs have approached steady state and maximum analgesic effect. Exceptions to this rule are:

- Continuous opioid infusions take 20 hours to reach steady state and should be adjusted once daily
- Transdermal fentanyl can take up to 48 hours to reach peak effect and should be adjusted every 3 days
- Methadone can take 3 to 5 days to reach steady state and should be adjusted weekly

Monitoring Administration Devices

Nurses have a responsibility to evaluate the accuracy of programming, integrity, and proper use of devices that administer analgesia (i.e., IV lines, epidural, or PCA systems). Monitoring should take place at least every 4 hours and whenever there is a change in medication, dosing order, or patient's condition.

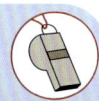

COACH CONSULT

Nurses use a variety of nondrug interventions to target different aspects of pain. Body-focused interventions, such as adjusting the bedding, repositioning, or massage; and applying lotions, ice, or heat packs to reduce the transduction and transmission of pain signals. Interventions that change the perception of pain include distraction, imagery, and cognitive reframing. Facilitating communication, problem-solving, and coping helps the patient reduce the underlying triggers of pain and suffering.

Monitoring for Side Effects

Like analgesics, adjuvant drugs should be administered in a consistent manner, with vigilant monitoring for adverse effects within the first hour after the initial administration at a particular dose. In contrast, NSAIDs need additional monitoring over time to detect damage to the renal, cardiovascular, and gastrointestinal systems that may develop silently after weeks, months, or years of therapy.

Providing Nondrug Interventions

In addition to pharmacological interventions, nurses provide nondrug interventions to relieve pain and provide comfort. Health-care organizations and state regulations vary greatly in which nondrug comforting measures nurses can implement independently. Ideally, interventions should attempt to interrupt the pain signal at the tissue, spinal, and brain levels simultaneously. For example, after knee surgery, ice may be applied to the joint, which is positioned for good alignment and comfort, while the patient listens to music that has personal meaning.

Back massages, which used to be part of routine evening nursing care, have recently been shown to reduce pain just after the massage and throughout the next day [12]. Other interventions that help alleviate pain are [13]:

- Music
- Guided imagery
- Relaxation
- Distraction
- Energy-based therapy (e.g., Reiki [14])
- Patient education
- Caring presence
- Reducing fear, anger, and anxiety

Responsibility to Evaluate and Refine the Treatment Plan

After implementing the plan, nurses must evaluate the safety and efficacy of each intervention. The plan is then refined based on individual responses and changing needs.

Efficacy

Evaluate the treatment plan accordingly, using the following criteria of efficacy:

- Reduction in pain intensity by at least 30% to 50%
- Improvement in patient's comfort, functioning, and satisfaction
- Facilitation of other treatment goals, such as:
  - Ability to tolerate therapy and procedures (e.g., dressing changes)
  - Ability to turn, cough, and deep breathe
  - Increase in ambulation distance
  - Duration of uninterrupted sleep

Safety

Monitoring for Sedation

In addition to efficacy factors, nurses evaluate the safety of the analgesic regimen. Most important is the identification of sedation and determining if it is related to an opioid. If doses of opioids exceed that which is needed for pain relief, the patient becomes sedated and respirations can be depressed. This most often occurs at the time of peak effect of the first dose or during a period of rapid-dose escalation. Sometimes a patient is alert while receiving high-dose opioids during a painful procedure. When the procedure is over and pain is reduced, the patient can become dangerously sedated. The nurse should monitor patients frequently after procedures for this possible occurrence.

Monitoring for Other Adverse Effects

Opioids produce constipation and usually require a stimulant laxative to reverse that effect. NSAIDs can produce silent gastrointestinal bleeding, elevate blood pressure, and reduce renal functioning. Older adults are particularly vulnerable to these effects and should be monitored periodically to rule out these problems. When patients have infusion pumps or other technologies to help treat their pain, nurses also must monitor for device-related complications (e.g., infiltrated lines, epidural hematoma).

Discharge Planning and Documentation

As the patient approaches discharge and analgesic doses are tapered, the patient may want information about nondrug pain relief methods, especially those that can be self-initiated at home. Perhaps the most important element of evaluating and refining the treatment plan is how the nurse ensures continuity of care. The clarity and completeness of the documentation and direct communication with other members of the treatment team is a vital, but often overlooked step in ensuring treatment success.

Nursing Role as an Interdisciplinary Team Member and Patient Advocate

Beyond direct patient care, nurses collaborate with and coordinate the plan of care in conjunction with the physician, other health-care providers, and family members [15]. The importance of nurse's role may be overlooked by other professionals [16] and policy makers. Nurses make a positive contribution by assertively communicating their opinions and observations about the patient's needs and responses.

Nurses also fulfill an important role as patient advocates. Often nurses develop an understanding of what the patient values, especially with regards to proposed medical interventions and possible outcomes. When

---

🗩 NURSE-TO-NURSE TIP

Stimulant Laxatives. Using a stimulant laxative, with or without stool softeners, can counteract opioid-induced constipation. However, providing a stool softener without a stimulant laxative creates what our palliative-care colleagues call "the mush without the push." Adding a bulking agent will only make the situation worse. Ironically, the misguided rationale for withholding a stimulant laxative is to avoid cramping, which happens when an enlarging stool mass sits in a hypoactive bowel.

patients fail to speak up or are not present when important treatment planning decisions are made, the nurse gives voice to the patients' perspectives, values, and preferences.

The Nurse's Role in Ethical Conflicts

Ethical conflicts arise when disagreements over potentially life-altering treatment occur (see Box 1–2). Common conflict types include:

- Autonomy vs. paternalism—patient and professionals want different things
- Beneficence vs. nonmaleficence—the most effective treatment may be harmful
- Autonomy vs. beneficence—patient refuses a clearly beneficial treatment
- Justice vs. nonmaleficence—treating people equally may be harmful based on individual vulnerabilities

In these cases, merely supporting the patient's right to autonomy does not resolve the ethical dilemma. When the nurse recognizes that conflicts exist, they have an ethical duty to begin conversations with involved parties.

The Nurse's Ethical Duty

Nurses are obligated to provide clinically competent and ethically defensible patient care. When ethical dilemmas exist, nurses facilitate team meetings and serve as patient advocates. Although nurses lack the authority of either physician or patient, they are uniquely situated to coordinate and initiate crucial conversations that can prevent or solve ethical problems. Getting involved parties together to engage in meaningful dialogue often has a positive long-term affect. When faced with these difficult circumstances, nurses should use all available resources, including:

- A trusted mentor
- Clinical nurse specialists or others with expertise pertinent to the situation
- Institutional ethics committees or ethics consultation services
- Relevant clinical and ethics literature [17–18]

THE ETHICS OF MORPHINE USE

The ethical double-effect principle is often given as a reason why strong analgesics, such as morphine, should not be used, despite severe pain. The implication that the benefits of morphine are negated by the potential harm it can cause should be challenged on clinical and ethical fronts. First, the intent of administering morphine, to relieve pain and suffering, is clinically and morally good. Second, pain can be relieved without harming the patient, by using proper administration and monitoring techniques. Finally, the failure to provide effective analgesia can be harmful and violates the patient's right to pain control.

Nursing Accountability to Relieve Pain

As health-care consumers become more sophisticated, they reject the notion that pain should be endured and are less reluctant than previous generations to use the civil court system when their rights to pain management are violated [19]. Although there have been cases brought against physicians for the undertreatment of pain, medical boards have acknowledged the failure but declined to take action against doctors.

Nurses are held legally accountable for inadequate pain care, as demonstrated in the following examples:

- The estate of an elderly man was awarded $15 million because of the needless suffering he endured when nurses administered placebos or weak analgesics for metastatic bone pain instead of morphine [20].
- The mother of an adolescent who received a placebo (saline instead of morphine) in an emergency room filed grievances against the prescribing physician and three nurses; disciplinary action was taken only against the nurses, who lost their licenses [21].

These cases and numerous others show that following doctors' orders does not absolve nurses from their professional duties.

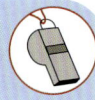

COACH CONSULT

Why are nurses more liable for placebo use than doctors? The guiding principle for medicine is, "above all else, do no harm." Central tenets for nurses involve respecting patients' dignity and autonomy while protecting them from incompetent, unethical, or impaired professional practice. Also, when determining liability, legal authorities consider the proximate cause. The nurse who administers a placebo is more directly involved in harming the patient than the doctor who wrote the order.

2009 Joint Commission Standards

Regulators require health-care organizations promise all patients they will attend to pain relief as a basic right. According to the 2009 Joint Commission standards, nurses need to know that:

- All patients have the right to pain management
- All patients must be screened for pain on arrival, and after any procedure requiring sedating or pain-relieving medications
- All patients who report pain need an in-depth pain assessment
- All patients who report pain must be treated or referred for treatment

In addition, all nurses need to:

- Be educated/oriented to their role in assessing and managing pain
- Conduct and document a pain assessment on all patients
- Follow safety procedures whenever administering high-alert medications for pain
- Evaluate and document the effect after each intervention for pain

Beyond the Basics

As nurses develop expertise and proficiency, they can progress from the role of novice in pain management to expert levels of practice. A growing number of advanced practice nurses specialize in pain management.

Pain Management Nurse

The standards of practice for pain management nurses parallel the nursing process, while the standards of professional performance detail the importance of [22]:

- Evaluating, role modeling, and promoting high quality of pain management practice
- Advancing one's own knowledge and competency in the specialty area
- Self-evaluating one's practice against regulations, guidelines, and best practices
- Collegiality to elevate the practice of peers and colleagues
- Collaborating with patients, families, and others to improve pain control
- Using ethics, research, and available resources to provide optimal care
- Promoting access and quality of care

One model of educating pain management nurses is through a *Pain Resource Nurse* program that has been developed and refined at various sites across the country [23]. This model has demonstrated significant improvements in the knowledge skills and attitudes regarding pain. Clinical outcomes (i.e., patient satisfaction and lower pain) and job satisfaction indicators improve with formal roles established for pain management nurses who undergo this training.

Advanced Practice Roles

Increasingly, nurses are practicing in expanded roles that have far-reaching responsibilities for managing the pain of individuals or groups of patients. Although nurse midwives and nurse anesthetists have important roles in managing their patients' pain, discussion here is limited to the nurse practitioner (NP) and clinical nurse specialist (CNS) roles.

Nurse Practitioner

The NP in pain management functions independently and interdependently in assessing and managing both medical and nursing problems related to pain [22]. Specifically, the pain management NP:

- Focuses on preventing pain and discouraging patients from worsening their condition
- Conducts a comprehensive pain assessment (i.e., history, physical, psychosocial, and spiritual)
- Orders diagnostic tests to aid in differential diagnosis
- Establishes and refines treatment plans based on practice model
- Educates and counsels patients with pain and their families

NPs have some degree of prescriptive authority in all 50 states and the District of Columbia, although there are restrictions on their prescribing of controlled substances in many states [24].

Clinical Nurse Specialist

The CNS in pain management supports nurses and nursing care of patients with pain, while emphasizing a multidisciplinary, multimodal approach to pain management [22]. The pain management CNS:

- Designs, implements, and evaluates pain programs and services
- Serves as a leader, resource, consultant and change agent (clinical or programmatic)
- Educates multidisciplinary clinicians, patients, and families using multiple methods
- Identifies opportunities for conducting and using research on pain
- Leads quality assessment and quality improvement activities

- Informs the public about pain via public relations, publications, and civic activities
- Develops educational programs, internal and external to the organization
- Consults with patients and professionals to provide optimal pain control

The CNS is less likely to have prescriptive authority than the NP, and there is considerable variation in regulations from state to state. There is some overlap in the roles and activities of the NP and the CNS, and some advanced practice nurses are certified in both roles. These nurses are uniquely qualified to provide comprehensive, effective, compassionate, and cost-effective care for a population many colleagues struggle to care for.

This handbook will provide the student or novice nurse with a clear understanding of the nurse's duty to manage pain and the skills to do so. This book simplifies complex theories to help the nurse understand the needs of patients with pain, assess pain across the life span, and plan comprehensive nursing care.

The focus throughout is on providing comfort. Even the novice nurse can comfort the most difficult patient by listening, believing, offering help, and providing explanations to the best of his or her ability. Even if an x-ray, blood test, or consultation with a specialist cannot identify the problem, pain is real. Nurses can always offer their caring presence, a distraction from pain, and comforting interventions.

WEB RESOURCES

A Google search of "Pain" yields more than 350 million hits. Some Web-based resources are helpful and reliable, while others are frighteningly misguided. A good starting point for credible pain information is:
- **Medline Plus:** http://www.nlm.nih.gov/medlineplus/pain.html
- **American Pain Foundation:** http://www.painfoundation.org
- **American Society for Pain Management Nursing:** http://www.aspmn.org/index.htm
- **Pain Treatment Topics:** http://pain-topics.org/

The art and science of pain management nursing is advancing at an incredible pace. Although we may not be able to eliminate pain today, we can almost always help the patient to think, feel, and do better. New treatments being developed today will make possible a more comfortable future.

2 The Nature of Pain

CHAPTER 2

The Nature of Pain

Pain is one of the most pervasive and expensive health-care problems of the 21st century [1–3], as:

- One-quarter of Americans have at least a full day of pain each month
- 45 million Americans have surgical pain each year with 80% experiencing severe pain during their recovery (mostly preventable by knowledgeable, attentive care)
- More than 20 million Americans have arthritis, the leading cause of disability
- 60% of older adults with pain have endured it for more than a year, and 20% of older adults receive no treatment for pain
- Pain is the second most common cause of workplace absenteeism costing industry nearly $100 billion each year in productivity and replacement costs
- 10% of patients have pain-related disability a year after surgery or trauma

Despite remarkable progress in prevention, diagnosis, and therapy, the incidence of pain is increasing, as are the challenges of easing it. Because of its increasing prevalence, high-economic costs, and negative affect on quality of life of patients and their families [4], uncontrolled pain is a public health priority. To treat pain effectively, nurses need to understand its true nature, a concept that scholars have long debated.

Historical Views of Pain

Throughout history, beliefs about the nature of pain have evolved from being a purely mystical or spiritual phenomenon; to being viewed as an emotional state; to being an entirely physical state. Current thinking views it as a multidimensional phenomenon, which nurses need to understand to provide optimal, effective multimodal therapy.

Ancient Thinkers

Since the beginning of recorded history, every generation has struggled to understand and deal with pain. The Old Testament's account of Adam and Eve describes pain as punishment for temptation and disobedience. Other ancient text and art depicts pain as having evil or mystical origins. The word "pain" is derived from the Greek *POINE* (goddess of revenge) and the Roman *POENA* (spirit of punishment). In some traditions, pain could be relieved only by penance, self-improvement, or meditation.

The virtues of controlling pain throughout history have been depicted in several ways. God put Adam in a deep sleep to remove a rib. Later, Hippocrates gave women willow bark instead of the more harmful, popular pain treatments of the day [5]. Many ancient strategies were designed to drive out the evil root of pain. These included:

- Craniotomy (ranging from piercing to stoning)
- Sucking evil out of the body (piping, cupping)
- Driving evil out by applying electric eels, pressure, or heat
- Using herbs or poisons (sometimes to induce coma or trances)
- Participating in mystical rites and ceremonies

Early Scientists and Philosophers

Although classical Greek philosophers Plato and Aristotle debated opposing views on most topics, they did agree, that pain was an emotional state. They envisioned human emotion as a continuum, with pleasure and ecstasy at one end and pain and suffering at the other. These thinkers dismissed the notion that pain was a deity-dispensed form of punishment for wrongdoing. They moved the basis of pain from a spiritual phenomenon (the soul) to the heart, which was long known as the center for sensations and emotion. Almost 2 millennia later, Leonardo da Vinci retained the notion of pain and pleasure as polar opposite emotions; however, he believed that sensations from the heart traveled along the nerves, via the spinal cord, to the third ventricle of the brain [5].

One hundred fifty years later, in the mid-17th century, Rene Descartes redrew one of da Vinci's drawings to emphasize the mechanistic and completely physical nature of pain pathways. He argued that when you stick your foot in fire, it opens the pores and tugs on a cord that rings a bell in the brain ventricles. As the bell swings back the other way, it tugs on the cord, pulling the foot out of fire before the person has a chance to respond emotionally to the experience (see Fig. 2–1). This drawing differed from

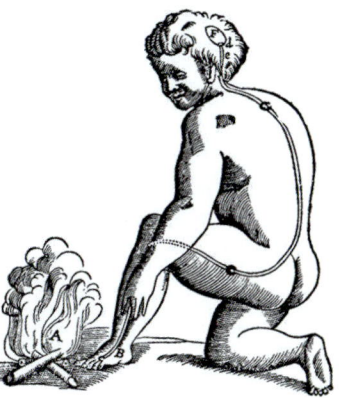

FIGURE 2–1: Rene Descartes' offer of proof that pain was purely physical: Fire contracts a cord, drawing the bell-like mechanism within the brain to one side. As it swings back into place it pulls the foot out of fire before awareness and emotional response occurs.

da Vinci's by removing the pathway through the heart. This shift moved the basis of pain from the heart (emotional center) to the brain (center of bodily functions). This drawing also formed the basis of **specificity theory** that specific physiological structures, rather than emotions or spirits explained the experience of pain. The specificity theory stimulated 400 years of productive research mapping nervous system details [6].

Modern Scientific Thought

By the middle of the 20th century, the inadequacies of Descartes' specificity theory were apparent. Specificity theory could not explain:

- Certain types of pain (e.g., phantom limb pain)
- Severely injured people who deny feeling pain

 WHY IS DESCARTES IMPORTANT?

Descartes' contribution inadvertently produced the so-called split between mind and body: the mistaken assumption that pain can either be physical or mental, not both. Pain that exists without physical explanations represents a mental defect. Conversely, if a patient is experiencing physical pain, his or her emotional state may be overlooked. Remember: an absence of evidence is not *evidence of absence*; it is merely evidence of limited technology. Also bear in mind that the mind and body are connected, and pain exists in both.

- The tremendous variation in pain perception in the same individual at different times
- How pain can persist or return even after pain fibers are cut

The competing **pattern theory** accounted for abnormal pain states as products of the summation of nerve inputs or a repatterning within the central nervous system (CNS). By 1960, Livingston and Noordenbos advanced the concepts described in the 19th century by Goldscheider detailing how pathological pain resulted from a repatterning of the peripheral, autonomic, and CNS. Specific sensory end organs or pain pathways were less important than the sum of all inputs at any given time or the changes that occur in the structure and function of the nervous system over time [7]. Although the pattern theory explained pathological pain states well, it was inconsistent with anatomical and physiological facts regarding how pain is processed in healthy individuals.

Other theoretical approaches to understanding and treating pain from a psychological perspective echoed Aristotle's notion that pain is an emotional state. Modern approaches added cognitive factors (e.g., hypochondria) and behavioral factors (e.g., personality disorder) to explain pain. Many of these theories describing pain as a purely psychological state were discredited in the late 20th century when research demonstrated that there was no such thing as a pain-prone personality and that chronic pain precedes depression rather than being a manifestation of mental illness [8,9].

Linkages between pain and learned responses have been studied. Pavlov's famous dog studies supported the view that responses to pain can be a learned phenomenon. He demonstrated that pain's meaning could be changed through operant conditioning, so that dogs could learn to salivate in eager anticipation of a steak whenever pain was felt [7].

 WHY IS PATTERN THEORY IMPORTANT?

Pattern theory emphasized the role of impulse intensity and patterns of nerve firing as causing pain. One pattern, central summation, intensifies pain as different stimulation types bombard the nervous system. This explains why bright, noisy environments worsen headaches. Temporal summation occurs when repeating the same stimulation (e.g., a pinprick) over time is perceived as being more painful because peripheral nerves become irritated and more sensitive. Prolonged excitation produces neuroplastic changes that spread and prolong pain.

The greatest puzzles and lessons about pain during the 20th century came about as a result of World War II. Astute clinicians caring for the wounded on the battlefield repeatedly observed patients who denied feeling pain and refused analgesia, despite extensive injuries. These same soldiers would then have robust pain responses to preoperative penicillin injections. This prompted the widely pondered question, "How can a shot hurt worse than being shot?" Devoted to seeking an answer to this question, two field surgeons, Patrick Wall and John Bonica, began focusing on the problems of understanding and treating pain (respectively). Bonica advanced practice when he developed the first interdisciplinary pain clinic in 1947 to help veterans with persistent pain. Later he laid the foundation for scientists and clinicians around the world to solve the puzzles of pain by forming the International Association for the Study of Pain (IASP).

COACH CONSULT

Nurses should avoid giving subtle but powerful messages to patients that rely on outdated notions about pain. For example, negative responses to reports of pain (e.g., What did you do? Didn't you follow our instructions?), suggest that pain is a punishment for wrongdoing. Suggesting that there is nothing wrong on the x-ray, so a patient's pain must be "in the head" conveys the mistaken belief that pain either has to be physical or mental, not both.

Patrick Wall, researching neurophysiologic mechanisms, teamed with Ronald Melzack, who studied behavioral aspects of pain. They shared their insights and articulated the **gate control theory** of pain in 1965. This theory states that pain perception is influenced by multiple biological, psychological, and social factors [10]. A shot could hurt worse than being shot because a barrage of physical, mental, and emotional factors facilitated transmission of the injection pain while blocking that of a nonlethal wound. Since the gate control theory, there has not been a similar grand theory trying to explain all types of pain. Instead there is a growing appreciation for the complexity of pain and for the differences between various types of pain.

Types of Pain

The IASP defines pain as "an unpleasant sensory *and* emotional experience associated with actual *or* potential tissue damage, or described in terms of such damage" [11]. The reader's attention is directed to the italicized words (*and, or*) where emphasis was added to this definition to point out that pain is always sensory *and* emotional and it is present with *or* without identified tissue damage. Pain may be categorized by:

- Location
- Duration

- Intensity
- Underlying mechanism

The most common distinctions are based on duration (i.e., acute versus chronic) or mechanism (i.e., nociceptive versus neuropathic).

Pain Classified by Location

Classifications based on pain location (e.g., headache, backache, chest pain) may be useful in determining the patient's underlying problems or needs, or they may be confusing given that most patients do not fit neatly into a single category. For example, there are 300 recognized types of headaches, many with similar clinical presentations but different clinical needs [12]. Additionally, low-back pain or chest pain may be caused by a variety of conditions, some are life threatening while others are transient and benign. Complicating the labeling of pain by location is the fact that some pains radiate to adjacent areas, while other pains may be referred to distant parts of the body. For example, cardiac pain may be felt in the fingers or jaw, with or without chest pain.

Pain Classified by Intensity

Pain often is categorized by intensity. The simple descriptor scale, ranking pain as mild, moderate, or severe has long been used, but has increasingly been replaced with the numeric (0 to 10) rating scale. In a landmark, multinational study of cancer pain, a numeric pain rating was linked to health and functioning scores. Pain in the 1 to 4 range was deemed mild pain, 5 to 6 was moderate pain, and 7 to 10 was graded as severe pain based on functional and health outcomes [13]. Because moderate and severe pain produced physical, mental, and social harm, keeping pain below the midpoint on the pain scale (≤4/10) often is used as a benchmark for successful treatment.

Pain Classified by Duration

The most common way to categorize pain is based on its duration:

- **Acute** or **transient pain** lasts seconds, minutes, hours, or days.
- **Chronic pain** lasts for months or years.

The category of **subacute pain** sometimes is used to indicate whether pain is prolonged beyond the normal healing time, but less than the cut point (3 or 6 months) established for chronic pain. From a nursing diagnosis perspective, there is only acute or chronic pain [14].

- Acute Pain: severe discomfort with a duration of less than 6 months
- Chronic Pain: severe discomfort with a duration of more than 6 months

Pain Classified by Mechanism

Pain may be classified as nociceptive or neuropathic:

- **Nociceptive pain** is experienced when an intact, properly functioning nervous system sends signals that tissues are damaged, requiring attention and proper care. Subcategories of nociceptive pain include:
  - **Somatic pain** originates in the skin, muscles, bone, or soft tissue. The somatic nerves are highly organized so character, intensity, and location of perceived pain is closely aligned with the type and extent of the injury.
  - **Visceral pain** results from activation of specialized (pain or autonomic) fibers that innervate organs and hollow viscera in a variable manner. Visceral pain thus tends to be poorly localized, and may have a cramping, throbbing, pressure or aching quality. Visceral pain often is associated with diaphoresis or nausea. Examples include labor pain, angina pectoris, and migraines.
- **Neuropathic pain** is experienced by people who have damaged or malfunctioning nerves, and is sometimes referred to as *pathological pain*. The nerves may be abnormal due to illness (painful diabetic neuropathy), injury (spinal cord injury), or undetermined reasons. Neuropathic pain is classified further as peripheral or central:
  - **Peripheral neuropathies** (e.g., postherpetic neuralgia) follow damage and/or sensitization of peripheral nerves
  - **Central neuropathic pain** (e.g., spinal cord injury, poststroke pain) results from damaged/malfunctioning nerves in the CNS. Some cases of neuropathic pain may result from failure to treat pain in an expedient, effective manner and therefore might have been preventable during the acute or subacute phases [15].

Three other types of pain occasionally referred to are: inflammatory pain, cancer pain, and sympathetically maintained pain. **Cancer pain** is

> **COACH CONSULT**
>
> Can you guess the likely pain type based on your patient's description of the pain? Among nociceptive pain types, pain described as "pinching" is likely to be somatic, while "cramping" more often describes visceral pain. Neuropathic pain commonly is described as "burning," "shooting" (peripheral), or "tingling" (central). A description of "intolerable" is most commonly used for chronic pain, whereas "discomfort" is used to describe acute pain.

well studied and includes pain directly related to the tumor, specific pain syndromes, and treatment-related sources of pain. Approximately 30% of patients newly diagnosed, nearly 50% of patients undergoing treatment and 70% to 90% of patients with advanced cancer experience pain. The principles of treating cancer pain, such as the analgesic ladder described in the pharmacology chapter, have been long accepted. Sadly, 26% of cancer patients over age 65 who experience daily pain, do not receive any analgesic agent [19].

Inflammatory pain results from a chemical buildup of irritants associated with tissue damage and inflammation. These chemicals sensitize nerves and facilitate the transduction and transmission of pain. When tissues are inflamed, redness, swelling, and pain rapidly escalates. When nerves are inflamed, pain also flares, while structural and functional neurological changes take place, setting the stage for chronic neuropathic pain to develop.

Sympathetically maintained pain may occur when abnormal connections develop between pain fibers and the sympathetic nervous system. Alpha-adrenergic sensitivity also may occur, so that spontaneous pain develops at times of noradrenaline release. The result is a perpetuation of problems with both the pain and sympathetically controlled functions (e.g., edema, temperature, and blood-flow regulation) that also tend to become chronic and neuropathic in nature.

A Fusion of Theories

Awaiting the articulation of a new grand theory to replace the gate control theory, current scholars in the field use concepts derived from past theories that have continued relevance and empirical support. Key relevant theories will be summarized, then key concepts synthesized as a framework for pain management nursing practice.

Summary of Key Theories

Key theories of pain significantly advanced our understanding of pain and the development of innovative therapies. They provide different lenses through which nurses can better understand patient's experiences and needs. Key theories include:

- **Specificity theory** contributed the idea of specialized receptors, fibers, nerve pathways, and other components of the sensory system.
- **Pattern theory** contributed the idea that changes in the spinal substantia gelatinosa, where sensitization and windup occur, account for pathological pain states [20].
- **Psychological and behavioral theories** contributed the ideas that affect, motivation, learning, perception, and central control play major roles in the pain experience.
- **Gate control theory** contributed the integration of theories listed above, to help explain physiological and pathological pain states and the wide range of individual responses to pain observed clinically. Key features of this theory focused on modulation of pain at the spinal dorsal horn, with inputs including:
  - Small afferent nerve (A-δ and C) fibers carry pain signals to the dorsal horn
  - Signals are modified by the substantia gelatinosa (influences excitatory or inhibitory state of spinal segment) before reaching proximal nerve ending
  - At the spinal end of the peripheral nerve, a gate is encountered
    - Opened gates release chemical messengers of pain into the synapse
    - Closed gates prevent the transmission of pain
  - The gates can be opened or closed by multiple factors
    - Peripheral stimulation of touch/temperature fibers
    - Descending signals from different brain regions (e.g., affect, motivation, and centers that regulate nerve excitability)
    - Neurotransmitters (from multiple influences) in the dorsal horn

Gate control theory explains how "kissing a boo-boo" relieves pain. A superficial burn sends noxious impulse waves through opened dorsal horn gates to be perceived. The light touch, warm breath, and moist sensations from the kiss stimulate large fibers to close the pain gates. Descending mechanisms activated by feelings of love, lessened fear, or motivation to stop crying also suppress the excitability of spinal nerves, diminishing the gate's capacity to fully transmit pain impulses.

Limitations of Current Theories

Although each of the theories presented has merit in explaining some aspect of pain, all have some limitations. The gate control theory has been praised for its breadth and criticized for its simplicity. It has stimulated research, inspired discourse, and provided a framework for educating professionals about pain. Thirty years after its publication, authors Melzack and Wall have come to a different understanding about the nature of pain.

Ron Melzack believed that focusing only on the dorsal horn as the primary place where pain signals are modulated was a mistake. Instead, he has come to believe that modulation of pain occurs at every interneuronal junction, with multiple ascending, descending, and parallel nerve influences. Pain is ultimately a product of the brain, rather than the sum of spinal input. Melzack described the brain's neuromatrix as a fully integrated network that creates pain from multiple neurological levels. He retained many of the gate control influences, while adding concepts of stress regulation and action systems as contributors to the perception of pain [21].

Patrick Wall also moved away from viewing pain modulation as a gating mechanism limited to the dorsal horn. The notion of a gate mechanism implies that pain can be either stopped or allowed to pass. Instead, he preferred the concept of a gain mechanism. Borrowing from an electrical perspective, a **gain control mechanism** regulates the strength of electrical impulses allowed to pass. In this view, pain modulation is like a volume dial (gain control) rather than the on-off switch implied by a gate control (personal conversation 8/24/99). Wall also believed that amplifiers and dampeners of pain signals extended beyond the dorsal horn, beyond the neuromatrix, to include social and cultural influences [22].

A Framework for Practice: Pain Control Targets

Unfortunately, Patrick Wall died before formalizing a gain control theory. The author believes those concepts would have provided nurses with a better framework for understanding and treating all types of pain than currently exists. Even without a formal theory, the concepts implied are supported by research suggesting that nurses need to:

- Abandon the notion that a single spinal gate can turn pain on or off
- Acknowledge that multitiered factors are capable of amplifying or dampening pain
- Assess and manage pain in a way that addresses targets throughout the nervous system and biopsychosocial non-neuronal focal points

This approach unites important concepts from psychological and behavioral theories with those that are more biologically based. This is consistent with the belief that pain, thoughts, emotions, and behaviors are all related to the action of nerves. Nerves are always changing in response to internal and external stimuli that are perceptible or imperceptible. Thus stimuli originating in the body, mind, spirit, or social situation can amplify or dampen signals of pain. Figure 2–2 provides examples of factors at each level that can heighten or lower the intensity of perceived pain. Nurses can then target these factors to diminish pain by cutting its amplification and activating dampeners.

Body

Endogenous chemical mediators that amplify pain (e.g., glutamate, substance P, and prostaglandins) and inhibit pain (e.g., endorphins, and norepinephrine); and cellular changes affecting pain intensity are detailed in Chapter 3. Conditions that threaten tissue integrity, such as repetitive strain, inflammation, hypoxia, or infection, need expedient identification and treatment. Tension and either prolonged disuse or overexertion of muscles near the site of pain also can amplify its intensity. In contrast, the local application of ice, heat, rubbing, or electrical stimulation can diminish the pain in many cases.

Hormonal fluctuations, fluid/electrolyte imbalances, and acid/base imbalances can heighten pain sensitivity. Appropriate levels of exercise, adequate nutrition, hydration, and oxygenation produce optimal levels of endogenous opioids that diminish the amount of pain perceived. Muscle relaxation and paced activities can turn down the volume of muscular pain. Too much or too little sleep has been shown to amplify pain, whereas 6 to 9 hours of sleep per night are optimal for containing pain [23]. For some individuals, specific environmental factors, such as weather, lighting, or certain foods, are associated with higher or lower levels of pain.

Mind

Pain is an unpleasant experience that results in an uncomfortable mental state. The level of mental stress clearly influences its intensity, amplifying pain levels in many instances. In particular, longer duration and the accumulation of stressful demands magnify pain signals. Pain itself is a stressor that can impair memory and concentration, or cause delirium. Subsequent physical, emotional, cognitive, and behavioral coping that reduces stress also can affect pain and its consequences.

AMPLIFIERS OF PAIN

Spiritual
- Spiritual distress
- Sense of personal failure
- Lost connections to environment and community
- Dire meaning/suffering
- Energy unbalance

Social
- Socially isolated
- Relationship/role conflict
- Over-dependency
- Dysfunctional coping

Mind
- Emotional distress
- Sadness or anger
- Fear, worry, frustration
- High or prolonged stress
- Self doubts, helplessness
- Catastrophizing

Neurological
- Dermatone overstimulation
- Wind-up, sensitization
- Neuroplastic changes
- Neuronal inflammation
- Activation of microglia

Tissue
- Ongoing tissue damage
- Glutamate, substance P
- Prostaglandin, lactic acid
- Repetitive injury/strain
- Inflammation/infection
- Hypoxia
- Muscle tension/spasm

DAMPENERS OF PAIN

Spiritual
- Strong faith
- Essence of person unchanged
- Sustained, renewed sense of purpose
- Environmental/social contacts maintained
- Energy flow balanced

Social
- Socially engaging
- Meaningful, pleasurable activities pursued
- Effective communication
- Work, volunteering

Mind
- Emotionally stable, feel loved
- Self-efficacy, optimistic
- Acceptance, realistic appraisal
- Mental distraction
- Mindfulness
- Relaxation response

Neurological
- Dermatone stimulation (rubbing, heat, cold)
- Production/release of endorphins

Tissue
- Tissue repair, healing
- Tissue stimulation (rubbing, heat, cold, TENS)
- Optimal nutrition, oxygen
- Position support (brace)

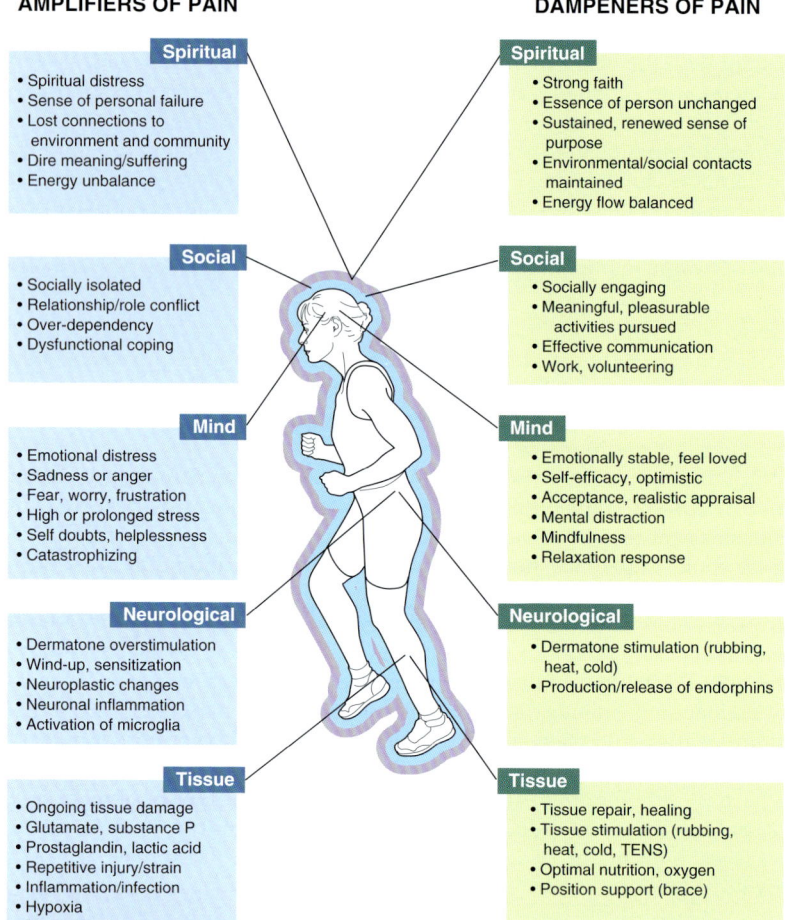

FIGURE 2–2: Pain control targets. Targets to help gain control of pain are present throughout the body, mind, spirit, and social interactions. Pain intensity can be lowered by reducing amplifiers and the use of dampeners.

Depressed mood or heightened anger, fear, and anxiety are known to cause an escalation of pain. Relaxation can decrease and counteract the effects of stress and may indirectly dampen pain. Feeling love, empathy, or joy and having either a good laugh or cry release endorphins that can diminish physical discomforts. Although emotions tend to fluctuate in a pattern that is closely associated with pain levels, the physical sensation of pain is not inextricably linked to emotional distress.

A person may have a high level of physical pain without distress, or may suffer emotional distress in the absence of pain. Although a distinct phenomenon, suffering is linked to pain in the following circumstances:

- Pain makes the person feel out of control
- The cause of pain is unknown
- The meaning of the pain is dire (e.g., associated with untreatable disease)
- The pain overwhelms the person
- The pain will likely never stop [24]

Especially when pain is severe or sudden, it stimulates the brain in a way that demands attention. Motivational factors and coping styles influence how this attention affects the perception and response to pain. Generally, focusing attention on pain can heighten the perceived intensity, just as distracting attention away from the pain can diminish it. Amplification of pain is likely not attributed to attention alone, as those who practice mindful meditation can learn to reduce pain by focusing attention on the sensation without allowing emotions or thought patterns to worsen pain [25].

Certain thought patterns are associated with pain levels. Strong self-doubts (i.e., low self-efficacy), unrealistic expectations, anticipation of high pain levels, rumination, learned helplessness, and cognitive distortions (e.g., magnification or catastrophizing) can contribute to treatment failures and escalate pain, disability, and depression [26–28]. In contrast,

 WHY IS STRESS SO IMPORTANT?

Stress occurs at various levels of intensity and on a continuum ranging from the good *eustress*, associated with valued achievements, to *distress*, associated with physical or mental harm. When stress is prolonged or at a moderately high level, the perception of pain is increased. However, at the most extreme stress levels, a person may be unaware of pain. Many anecdotes describe athletes performing superbly, or trauma victims rescuing others, apparently unaware of their painfully broken bones.

acceptance of pain, realistic expectations, and higher self-efficacy beliefs (i.e., confidence in one's ability to manage pain, function, and cope) are associated with lower pain levels, better clinical outcomes, and improved quality of life [29–30].

Spirit
The spirit comprises a person's innermost concerns and values, including the perceived purpose, meaning and driving force of life. Spiritual pursuits may include rituals that help the individual become part of a community, or feel a bond with nature or the universe. Severe or prolonged pain permeates the very essence of the person, eroding what is important and often challenging established beliefs and values [31–32]. In some spiritual or religious traditions, pain is viewed as a punishment for wrongdoing, or an opportunity to demonstrate their strength of character that will be rewarded after death. From this perspective, a person can willingly endure severe pain without suffering.

Spirituality is not limited to the confines of religious traditions. Some holistic frameworks view humans as irreducible energy fields in continual interaction with universal sources of energy. From this perspective, pain may be intensified or lessened as a result of changes in energy patterns. Therapeutic touch, Reiki, and acupuncture are examples of restorative modalities designed to improve energy-flow patterns to improve healing and lessen discomfort.

Social Situation
When pain is severe or chronic, it can lead to a withdrawal from social activities and contact with family, acquaintances and friends [33]. The resultant social isolation can worsen pain. Pain and suffering can be intensified further when there are hardships related to finances, role fulfillment, and intimacy. Patients with a family history of pain or a personal history of physical or sexual abuse are particularly vulnerable to heightened sensitivity to pain [34–40]. The presence of a caring person helps lower the intensity of pain, whereas aggressive or overprotective encounters may adversely affect pain severity. In contrast, improving the quantity and quality of relationships and resuming active roles within the family and society can lessen pain and suffering. When pain persists or intensifies to the point of disability, patients are often accused of feigning their symptoms to shirk responsibilities. Cases of patients consciously faking pain (i.e., malingering) or unconsciously expressing physical pain when emotionally distraught (i.e., somatoform disorders) represent a small percentage of patients with pain.

Rather than assume that secondary gains are motivating pain behaviors, nurses should first consider a patient's secondary losses. Anguish over lost goals or unfulfilled desires may lead many to greater pain, disability, and depression. For those unable to work, volunteering has been shown to reduce these negative effects, in part by reducing isolation and restoring a sense of purpose and value [41].

Therapeutic encounters are a form of social interaction. In fact the **placebo effect** is a beneficial outcome resulting from a positive social interaction of a therapeutic nature. Clinicians can help improve the efficacy of pain-relieving interventions by being compassionate and thorough while conveying confidence in treatment and the treatment team. Awareness of one's own values and nonverbal communication style can help the nurse establish an optimal pain-reducing therapeutic milieu.

COACH CONSULT

Social responses to the person with chronic pain affect the perceived pain. Punishing responses (i.e., anger, disbelief or confrontational) to reports of pain can make it worse and deteriorate the quality of social interactions. Interestingly, solicitous responses (i.e., those who show excessive concern, support, and help) also amplify pain [28]. Distracting responses that involve the person in activities seem to best neutralize pain.

Multimodal Approaches

Many other theoretical models can be used to understand pain and guide treatment. In addition to the theories described, there are mid-range or practice-based theoretical models that address the undertreatment of pain [43], comfort theory [44], or the science of symptom management [45] that are especially useful. Two concepts that many of these theories share are those of multimodal approaches to pain and balance [46].

NURSE-TO-NURSE TIP

Placebos are inert pseudotherapies without benefit, while *placebo effects* are desirable consequences of therapy facilitated by professionals who establish rapport, impart confidence, and convey enthusiasm about the treatment. Use of placebos is legally indefensible and unethical, but are still commonly prescribed by doctors for patients in pain [42]. Nurses should *not* administer placebos outside of approved research projects. However, nurses *should* use the placebo effect by administering the best available treatments with confidence, enthusiasm, and compassion.

There is a growing appreciation that a multimodal approach to nursing care is needed that targets multiple factors affecting pain levels simultaneously. Nurses are typically quite adept at meeting the physiological needs of their patients, but may need to expand their skill set in reversing pain amplification attributed to emotions and unhelpful thoughts. The importance of establishing and maintaining a high-quality therapeutic milieu and taking time to understand the context of pain in the patient's life may not be as highly valued as accurately documenting intake and output; however, it is an important step in helping patients with pain think, feel, and do better. Throughout this book, examples of multimodal approaches are described as they pertain to pharmacological, technology-assisted, and nonpharmacological methods of controlling pain.

Multimodal therapy simultaneously targets different pain-amplifying mechanisms. In doing so, medication doses can be lowered (with a resultant lower risk of harm), while providing the patient with the opportunity to learn coping, self-management, and health-promoting techniques. Through a balanced approach, nurses can treat pain in a way that also improves functioning and enhances the quality of life.

3 Physiology of Pain

Physiology

CHAPTER 3

Physiology of Pain

Pain transmission and perception is complex because (1) the central nervous system (CNS) is fully integrated and dynamic; (2) each individual perceives pain differently; and (3) only a tiny proportion of the cells, chemicals, and receptors believed to have a role in pain are fully understood. This chapter is divided into three sections:

- The physiology of pain when the nociceptive (pain signaling) system is working properly
- The physiological effect of unrelieved pain
- The pathological mechanisms responsible for abnormal pain states or neuropathic pain

This is an area of intensive research, building on decades of rapidly expanding knowledge. New insights about pain and the changes it produces within nerves are challenging the validity of long-standing approaches to pain. Details about the mechanisms involved with pain have resulted in the development of new types of treatments, currently in the process of gaining U.S. Food and Drug Administration (FDA) approval. Understanding pain physiology provides the solid foundation needed to support sound nursing decisions.

Physiology of Pain When Nociceptive System Works

The extent to which pain is perceived depends on dynamic interactions between nerves, other bodily systems and the environment. Nociceptive **pain** is experienced when a properly functioning nervous system sends signals that tissues are being exposed to potentially damaging conditions that require attention and proper care. Most tissues are innervated by nociceptors, which are designed to detect potentially harmful physical, chemical, or thermal stimuli; and respond by sending pain signals. When the nociceptors detect a painful stimulus, they fire off an impulse that travels to the spinal cord and/or midbrain. From there, the pain message is conveyed to many different areas of the brain's cortex. The areas of the brain activated by these signals, combined with other concurrent factors influence the way pain is perceived. This process, called nociception, involves four primary steps:

- Transduction
- Transmission
- Perception
- Modulation

Transduction

Transduction is the first step in the experience of pain. Put simply, stimuli or tissue damage activates nerve endings or sensory neurons (in this case, nociceptors) in the peripheral nervous system. The nociceptors open sodium (Na^+) and/or calcium (Ca^{++}) channels, sparking an electrical impulse, which is conducted along the nerve.

The ultimate perception of pain depends in part upon the location of the nociceptors, the types of nociceptors affected, and the type of stimuli received. Nociceptors respond differently to different stimuli, depending on where they are in the body. For example, a scratch that would trigger pain in the eye's cornea would not hurt a finger.

The various kinds of nociceptors react differently to harmful stimuli. The primary nociceptors (see Fig. 3–1) include [1]:

- High-threshold thinly myelinated A-delta (rapid, sharp, localized pain)

 WHY IS THE ABILITY TO FEEL PAIN IMPORTANT?

Some people are born unable to feel pain. The underlying pathophysiology is unclear, but there appear to be different types of insensitivity. In one type, patients lack of voltage-sensitive sodium channels responsible for pain transduction. Another type results from an overproduction of endorphins, which allows them to feel pain only when given naloxone. In a third type, patients can perceive pain but are indifferent to it. All of these patient types with a diminished capacity or inability to sense pain are in danger of allowing serious illness or injuries to go undetected and untreated.

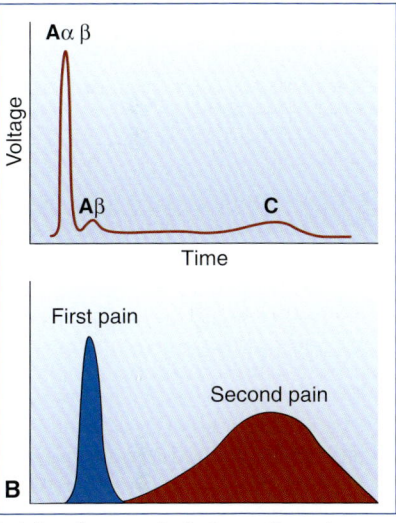

Primary Afferent Axons

Aα and Aβ fibers

Myelinated
Large diameter
Proprioception, light touch
Thermal threshold: None

Aβ fiber

Lightly myelinated
Medium diameter
Nociception
(mechanical, thermal, chemical)
Thermal threshold:
–53°C Type I
–43°C Type II

C fiber

Unmyelinated
Small diameter
Innocuous temperature, itch
Nociception
(mechanical, thermal, chemical)

A Thermal threshold: –43°C

Aα β

Voltage

Aβ   C

Time

First pain

Second pain

B

F I G U R E   3 – 1 : Sensory fiber types. *A,* Peripheral nerves include medium- to large-diameter A-alpha or A-beta (A,α,β) myelinated afferent fibers, small-diameter A-delta (Aδ) and small-diameter unmyelinated afferent C-fibers (C). *B,* Conduction velocity is directly related to fiber diameter, as demonstrated in the compound action potential recording from a peripheral nerve.

- High-threshold nonmyelinated C-fibers (slow, long lasting, dull, aching pain)
- Low-threshold well-myelinated A-beta (fast signals, touch, light breeze)

Compared with other sensory neurons, nociceptors are usually quiescent, have high activation thresholds, and conduct signals slowly toward the CNS [2].

Nociceptors can be classified based on the different types of stimuli they respond to:

- **Mechanoreceptors** sense trauma, pressure, cuts, twisting, pinching, etc.
- **Chemoreceptors** sense acids and inflamed, diseased, or ischemic tissue
- **Thermoreceptors** sense hot, burning, or cold

Some nerves are highly selective regarding the type of threats they will respond to, while others respond to multiple types of stimuli [3]. Different tissue types generally respond only to specific stimulus types [4]. For example:

- Skin responds to mechanical, thermal, and chemical threats
- Muscle (skeletal/cardiac) responds to chemical stimuli
- Joints respond to chemical or extreme mechanical threats
- Periosteum responds to mechanical stimuli
- Visceral tissue responds to chemical and specific mechanical (twisting, distention) threats

The intensity of the pain triggered depends upon the number and type of nociceptors activated, and their patterns of firing.

Transmission

The second step of nociception, transmission of pain, takes place after the electrical impulse has travelled the length of the peripheral nerve and enters the CNS. There, the signal must be transferred to other nerves for sensations or protective actions to occur. Here is how transmission works:

- The electrical impulses from peripheral nerves enter the spinal dorsal horn
- At the spinal dorsal horn, voltage-sensitive calcium channels open
- These channels trigger the release of neurotransmitters, aspartate and glutamate
- Aspartate and glutamate help trigger an impulse in projection neurons that extend to the midbrain, where the signal is relayed again to various higher brain centers

The nerve fibers stimulate projection neurons enough to overcome the calming effects of inhibitory interneurons, propelling message of the pain to the brain. The strength of this signal is determined by interacting factors affecting the excitability of the CNS (see Table 3–1).

Table 3–1	**Key Excitatory and Inhibitory Components of Pain (Normal State)**	
	COMPONENT	**DESCRIPTION**
EXCITATION		
By-products of tissue injury	Bradykinin, prostaglandins, histamine hydrogen ions, lactic acid	Sensitize nerves, lower activation threshold. Produce spontaneous activity. Activate acid-sensing channels. Increase membrane excitability.
Inflammatory products	TNF, interleukin	Irritate and sensitize nerves. Damage vulnerable receptors and nerves.
Neuron-produced peptides	Glutamate, CGRP, aspartate, substance P, cholecystokinin	Lower activation threshold, prolong discharge after stimulation (long-term potentiation). Cause sensitization of CNS.
	Serotonin (excitatory subtypes)	Irritate and sensitize peripheral nerves. Most types inhibit spinal transmission of pain. Subtype 3 initiates descending excitation responsible for windup of dorsal horn.
INHIBITION		
Neuron-produced peptides	GABA, glycine	Increase chloride ion entry to cell reduces nerve excitability, making it harder to generate action potentials.
	Serotonin, norepinepherine	Blocks calcium influx and release of excitatory neurotransmitters (aspartate and glutamate).
	Opioids	Prevent presynaptic opening of voltage-sensitive Ca^{++} ion channels needed for neurotransmitter release. Open postsynaptic K^+ channels. Activate descending inhibitory fibers that reduce nerve excitability.

TNF—tumor necrosis factor, CGRP—calcitonin gene-related peptide, GABA—gamma-aminobutyric acid.

There are a variety of factors that can lower the activation threshold of spinal nerves, leading to an amplified transmission of pain signals. As a result of enhanced transmission, pain is stronger and lasts longer than normal. Spinal factors that enhance transmission include:

- Higher concentrations of cations (Na^+ and Ca^{++} ions)
- Production and release of glutamate, the primary excitatory neurotransmitter
- Spinal inflammation by substance P, prostaglandins, and other products of inflammation
- Production and release of calcitonin gene-related peptide (CGRP)
- Production and release of nerve growth factor (NGF)

When strong enough signals reach the dorsal horn, they elicit a local response that activates reflexive responses, such as pulling your hand away from something hot. Projection neurons, if activated, transmit the signal of pain via specific tracts to higher centers, where it can be perceived (see Fig. 3–2).

The pain impulse is transmitted from the spinal cord to the brainstem and thalamus via three main nociceptive pathways: the spinothalamic pathway, the spinoparabrachial pathway, and the trigeminothalamic pathway. The **spinothalamic tract** is the most direct path to the ventral posterolateral nucleus (VPN), which connects to key cortical and subcortical brain centers. The **spinoparabrachial projections** transmit impulses through the reticular formation, pons, and hypothalamus before reaching the thalamic and higher pain centers. As for pain signals stemming from the head or face, the **trigeminothalamic tract** transmits them to the thalamus via the pons bypassing the spine.

Perception

Pain perception comprises the character, intensity, and meaning of pain to an individual. Interpretation of pain is influenced by psychological, social, and spiritual factors, and past experiences and future hopes. This interpretation influences an individual's behavioral responses. Three key factors influencing a person's perception of pain include:

- **Threshold:** the point at which the person identifies a particular stimulus as painful
- **Distractibility:** the degree to which the person can ignore the pain
- **Tolerance:** the point at which the person experiencing it acts to stop the pain

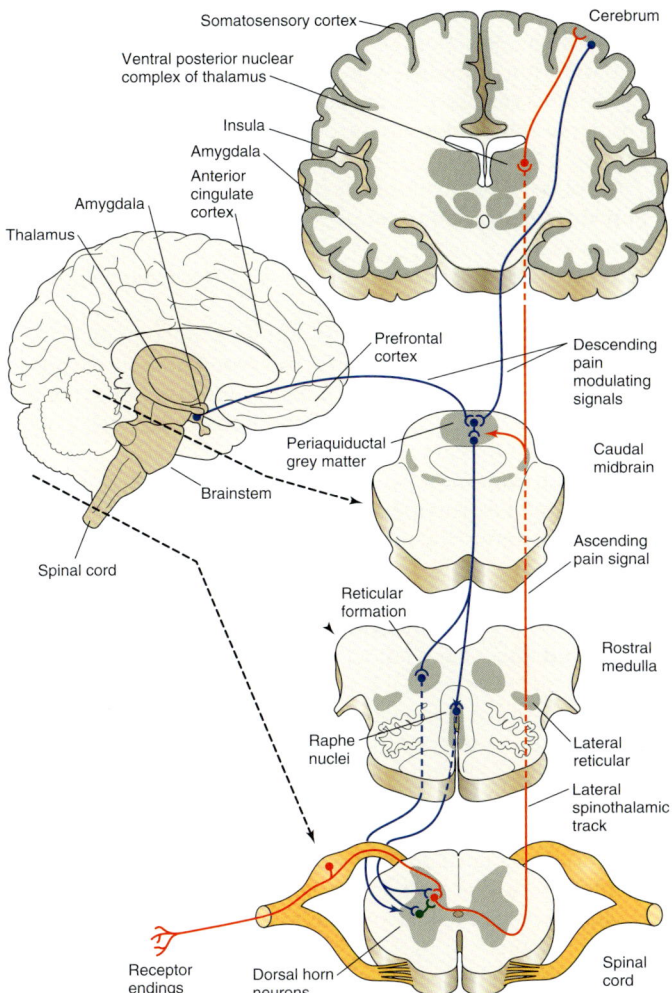

FIGURE 3–2: Pain-processing areas of the central nervous system. Common pain pathways are shown here: spinothalamic tract (red) crosses the dorsal horn to anterior, contralateral side; ascends to the thalamic ventral posterolateral nucleus (VPN). Descending modulating tracts (blue) influenced by cognitive, affective and motivational brain centers pass through the midbrain, reticular formation, and raphe nuclei to regulate ascending signal intensity.

Threshold and tolerance levels may vary based on the patient's focus of attention and thoughts about the cause or significance of the pain. A person whose attention is intensely focused elsewhere may be unaware of substantial injuries sustained. A person also may perceive pain even in the absence of nerve impulses from hurting parts of the body (e.g., phantom pain or post spinal cord injury pain) [5].

Pain perception is largely influenced by the sum of three distinct inputs:

- **Sensory/discriminative:** presence, location, intensity, quality of pain
- **Affective/motivational:** emotional distress and behavioral response
- **Cognitive/evaluative:** context and meaning of pain

Supporting that classification, pain is processed in multiple areas of the brain (see Table 3–2). A perception of higher intensity or sustained pain involves more areas of the brain and more intense neuronal activity. Subsystems of the brain that are activated by pain include:

- **Reticular system:** involves arousal and motivation that warn the person to attend to pain
- **Limbic system:** responsible for emotion, behavior, and long-term memory
  - **Insula** regulates subjective experiences, such as emotions and cravings, learning, motivation, and social responses
  - **Amygdala** attaches emotional significance to sensory inputs and handles emotional learning, moods, and memory; it also links cognitive areas with brainstem centers of pain modulation
- **Neuroendocrine system:** includes the hypothalamus, pituitary, and endocrine system that effects physical, emotional, and behavioral responses associated with pain

These brain regions are commonly activated by slow C-fibers, after the faster (A-delta) fibers have elicited a behavioral response. Patients often exhibit sudden, reflexive, behavioral reactions before they consciously perceive pain. Typical unconscious pain responses include [6]:

- Startle response
- Flexion of hurt body part (withdrawal) and postural readjustment
- Looking at, touching, or rubbing hurt area
- Adrenal (fight-or-flight) response
- Vocalizations (yell, moan, cry)

Two distinct brain centers (thalamus and sensory cortex) are believed to be essential for the perception of pain.

Table 3–2	**Key Dimensions and Structures Involved in Pain Perception**	
TYPE OF PERCEPTION	**ANATOMIC STRUCTURE**	**EFFECTS**
Affect/motivation	Reticular formation	Triggers arousal, alertness, aversive drive.
	Midbrain	Heightens reflexes, enhances learned behaviors.
	Limbic system	Causes anxiety, depression, or anger. Generates purposive actions and motivation.
	Hypothalamus	Integrates autonomic, neuroendocrine, emotional responses and motivation.
	ACC	Integrates affect (unpleasant feelings), cognition, and response selection.
	Insula	Produces learning, emotions, and memories related to pain.
Sensory/discriminative	Thalamus	Distinguishes features of pain and disseminates signals to facilitate discrimination of different sensations. Medial thalamus is concerned with affect and motivational aspects, while the lateral thalamus discriminates specific parts of sensory (character, location, intensity) pain.
	Sensory cortex	Discriminates the character, location, and intensity of pain.
	PAG	Initiates descending inhibitory signals from the brainstem to block pain in the dorsal horn.
Cognitive/evaluative	ACC	Integrates affect, cognition, and behavioral response selection.
	Cerebral cortex	Links sensory, motor, and association regions with important memory, perceptual awareness, thought, and language functions.

ACC—anterior cingulate cortex, PAG—periaqueductal gray.

Role of the Thalamus

The thalamus has a major role in pain processing, distributing information related to pain to different brain regions. Thalamic activity depends upon the signals it exchanges with the cerebral cortex and with the subcortical regions that regulate memory, motivation, coordination, and autonomic responses [5]. Specifically, the thalamus, amygdala, and insula mount an emotional and behavioral response; based on learning and memories.

Role of Higher Cortical Centers

Higher centers of the cortex integrate sensation, emotion, and thoughts amidst a context of past experiences, present focus, and future goals. This area of the brain allows individuals to assign meaning to the sensation of pain. The brain's primary sensation detector, the sensory cortex* (lateral postcentral gyrus of parietal lobe), quickly discerns details about the nature, intensity, and location of pain and other sensations. The cingulate cortex synthesizes this information, producing the overall perception of pain. The various sections of the cingulate cortex serve different functions:

- **Anterior:** executive functions, such as planning or problem-solving
- **Posterior:** evaluative functions
- **Dorsal:** cognitive functions
- **Ventral:** emotional functions

See the Coach Consult box for examples of how psychological factors can affect pain perception.

COACH CONSULT

Thoughts, feelings, motivation, and other psychological factors play an important role in the perception of pain. Pain often measures higher at night when distractions of the daytime are gone. Fear of needles will drive up pain and the motivation to escape injections. With chronic pain, a depressed mood and catastrophic thought patterns are associated with the perception of more pain. In contrast, athletes, intently focused on competition, may be unaware of pain.

Modulation

Modulation of pain often is described as the final step in nociception. **Modulation** refers to the increase or decrease in pain signal intensity that can occur before, during, and after pain is perceived. Pain can be dampened or amplified at every nerve junction, and influenced by physical, psychological, social, spiritual, and environmental factors.

When pain pathways are activated, a combination of nerve factors influence (modulate) the intensity of pain. Some nerve factors facilitate pain transduction and transmission in both central and peripheral neurons, such as substance P. These facilitators increase the perceived signal

---

*The term *sensory cortex* is used instead of *somatosensory cortex* in this text.

intensity. In contrast, endorphins dampen signal intensity by inhibiting pain transmission. Other nerve factors can have variable effects, such as norepinephrine, that excites peripheral nerves but inhibits central nerves.

Overall, three key modulation processes amplify, spread, and prolong pain: peripheral nerve sensitization, central nerve sensitization, and dorsal horn windup. In contrast, only one modulating process, the descending inhibitory systems, can reduce pain signal intensity.

Peripheral Nerve Sensitization

Potential or minor tissue damage does not produce strong enough signals to generate a pain impulse until inflammation of both tissues and nerves lower the activation threshold. In normal circumstances, inadvertently bumping one's hand against a table is not enough to hurt. However, if the local tissue and nerve was sensitized, by a recent burn, cut, or infection, pain from the same stimulus could be substantial. Peripheral nerve sensitization amplifies pain by any one, or a combination, of the following processes:

- Damaged tissues produce irritating chemicals
  - Bradykinin, histamine, serotonin, prostaglandins, leukotrienes, K^+, H^+
- Immune responses release additional vasoactive and irritating chemicals
  - Interleukins, interferon, NGF, tumor necrosis factor (TNF)
- Activated afferent fibers release other irritants at both ends of the nerve
  - Substance P, CGRP, neurokinin A, histamine, acetylcholine, bradykinin
- Tissue and neurogenic inflammation sensitize adjacent nerves (see Fig. 3–3)
- Peripheral nerves produce enzymes (cyclic AMP,* protein kinases) that:
  - Change ion-specific (sodium, potassium, and calcium) channel density
  - Lower the activation threshold
  - Strengthen the responses to stimuli
- Excess intracellular positive ions hyperpolarize nerves causing excessive, repeated firing
- Growth of new nerve endings that expand the receptive field of peripheral nerves
- Previously insensate (silent) nociceptors become active and signal pain

*Cyclic AMP refers to **Cyclic adenosine monophosphate.**

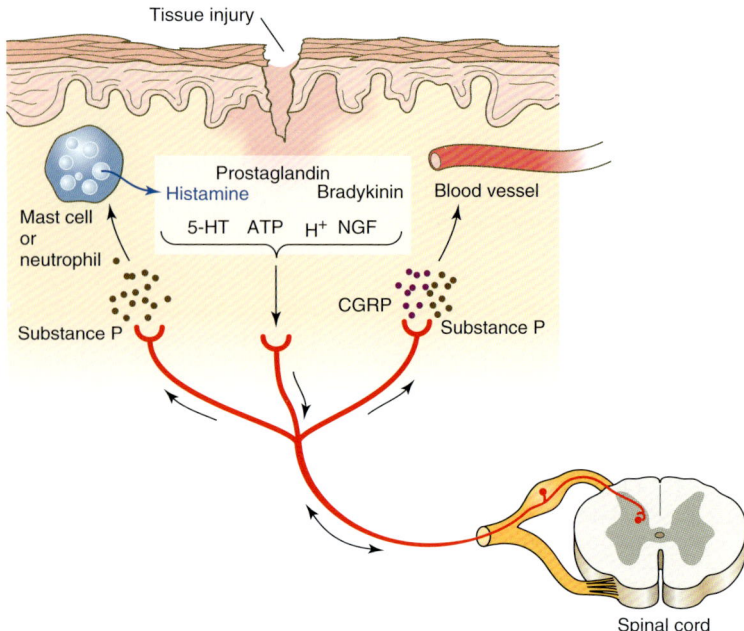

Tissue injury

Prostaglandin
Histamine   Bradykinin   Blood vessel

5-HT   ATP   H⁺ NGF

Mast cell
or
neutrophil •

Substance P   CGRP
                             Substance P

Spinal cord

FIGURE 3–3: Mechanisms of peripheral sensitization. Some of the primary components that sensitize peripheral nerves include peptides (bradykinins), lipids (prostaglandins), neurotransmitters (serotonin [5-HT and ATP]) and neurotrophins (NGF). Each of these factors sensitize (lower the threshold) or excite the terminals of the nociceptor by interacting with cell-surface receptors expressed by these neurons. Activation of the nociceptor not only transmits afferent messages to the dorsal horn but also initiates neurogenic inflammation by releasing neurotransmitters, notably Substance P and CGRP, from the peripheral terminal. This in turn, induces vasodilation and plasma extravasation (leakage of proteins and fluid from postcapillary venules), and activating non-neuronal cells, including mast cells and neutrophils. These cells then contribute additional irritants to the involved tissue and nerves.

Central Nerve Sensitization

Many of the same chemical mediators that sensitize peripheral nerves also enhance pain processing in the CNS (see Fig. 3–4).

Additional CNS factors that amplify pain include:

- Buildup of intracellular and extracellular cations (sodium and calcium)

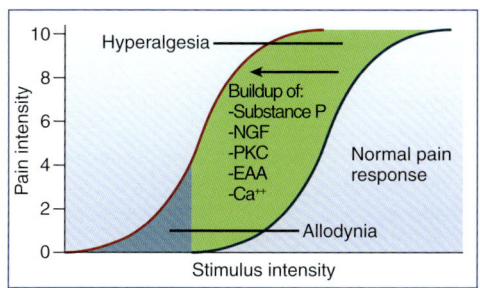

FIGURE 3–4: Effect of windup and central sensitization. This figure shows some of the more important factors associated with spinal sensitization and windup that amplify pain and set the stage for hyperalgesia and allodynia to develop. NGF—nerve growth factors, PKC—intracellular buildup of protein kinease-C, EAA—buildup of excitatory amino acids, Ca++—calcium ion buildup.

- Accumulation of excitatory amino acids (glutamate and aspartate)
- Neurogenic inflammation releases substance P, CGRP, and neurokinin
- C-fiber terminals in dorsal horn degenerate and low threshold A-beta fibers sprout to fill the void left by damaged C-fiber terminals
- Excitatory glial cells are activated, multiply, and release nerve irritants

These factors combine to produce hyperalgesia and allodynia.

COACH CONSULT

Keep in mind that as a person experiences pain, neurons develop a memory for it, resulting in a more rapid and efficient response to future pain. This heightens sensitivity to pain in previously hurt body parts.

Dorsal Horn Windup

The windup phenomenon was first described in animal experiments where the same electrical stimulus was observed to produce stronger pain when repeated. Windup occurs in people whenever repeated signals activate the spinal dorsal horn, a response is triggered by descending excitatory fibers, which produce primary and secondary hyperalgesia that strengthen and spread pain signals (see Box 3–1).

The windup phenomenon involves the following physiological changes [3]:

- Activation of nerves to release neurotransmitters that augment nerve excitability
- Wide dynamic range cells change their structure and function, thereby lowering the activation threshold and extending nerve sprouts into the dorsal horn that spread pain

- Glutamate-sensitive N-methyl-D-aspartate (NMDA) receptors multiply, triggering a release of the excitatory amino acid glutamate
- Sustained depolarization and low postsynaptic activation thresholds develop

When overwhelmed by excitatory amino acids, inhibitory nerves malfunction and eventually die, resulting in pathological changes in the CNS. Such changes to the CNS can yield strong, prolonged pain that no longer serves as a useful warning.

> **NURSE-TO-NURSE TIP**
>
> Windup phenomenon progressively facilitates pain so that when the same signals are repeated, they generate stronger and longer duration responses. This response produces primary hyperalgesia. As excitatory cells, receptors, and chemicals accumulate in the spine, adjacent nerves also become hyperexcitable, producing secondary hyperalgesia and spreading pain. Because repeated or continuous pain causes windup, it is important for nurses to prevent by treating pain before it intensifies and creates the physiological changes that magnify pain further.

Descending Inhibitory Mechanisms

Certain nociceptive stimuli activate descending inhibitory mechanisms capable of reducing pain. Key opioid-producing interneurons and opioid receptors are found throughout the CNS. These structures are normally abundant in the spinal dorsal horn, reticular formation, periaqueductal gray (PAG), hypothalamus, thalamus, cingulate cortex, and cerebral cortex. Descending inhibitory pathways run parallel to ascending pain signals, inhibiting pain signal transmission by different mechanisms, including:

- Gamma-aminobutyric acid (GABA) and glycine are primary inhibitory neurotransmitters affecting the flow of zinc and chloride ions to calm nerves
- Subtypes of serotonin and norepinephrine have inhibitory actions in the CNS
- Endogenous opioids (e.g., endorphins), act as morphine to block glutamate release, facilitate potassium (K^+) escape, and prevent the activation of pain transmitting nerves

The net effect is diminished or blocked transduction and transmission of pain signals.

Role of Psychosocial Factors

Psychosocial factors also may facilitate or inhibit perception of pain. Shortages of beta-endorphins in the CNS have elicited the following factors known to escalate pain:

- Fear
- Anxiety
- Depression
- Learned helplessness

Anticipation and/or expectation of pain enhances pain of every type, resulting in activation of pain circuits and heightened perception of pain

---

 ON THE HORIZON

The precise role of specific modulators remains unclear. Many are understood when isolated, but act differently in concert with each other. For example, neurotensin and dynorphin inhibit pain in some circumstances and amplify pain in others. Their physiological actions vary depending on the site of action, and whether or not the person is stressed or has chronic pain. When the interplay of these modulators is better understood, therapies can be designed to block their excitatory actions and enhance their inhibitory functions.

intensity. In contrast, anticipation of pain relief, as seen with placebo-induced analgesia, releases endorphins from the PAG and amygdale, and reduces perception of pain.

Stress can sometimes be good for pain reduction. Abrupt physical or emotional stressors may influence pain by increasing sympathetic nervous system (SNS) arousal and promoting endogenous opioid (endorphin) production. This phenomenon is known as **stress-induced analgesia**. At the same time, however, stress can make pain worse. Prolonged stress lowers endorphin, cortisol, and growth hormone levels in a way that increases pain, reduces healing capacity, and enhances vulnerability to illness [7, 8]. In an acutely stressful situation, such as trauma, a patient may not feel pain associated with significant injury. Health professionals must thoroughly assess these patients even if they deny pain. In contrast, prolonged stress must be managed to promote comfort, health, and healing.

Effect of Unrelieved Pain

Despite scientific and professional advances in pain control, needless pain and suffering is still common in many health-care settings. See Chapter 1 for a review of the professional, patient, and system-related barriers or mistaken beliefs that undermine effective pain treatment. Poorly managed pain can result in many problems, not only for patients but also for health-care organizations, including patient dissatisfaction, prolonged institutionalization, readmissions, and increased costs [8]. Unrelieved pain undermines goals of health care by interfering with: healing, immunity, and function [8, 9]. Because pain interferes with healing and immunity, unrelieved pain also puts patients at risk for developing complications. It can harm all body systems. Potential problems that may arise from unrelieved pain include:

- Lowered ejection fractions of patients with left ventricular dysfunction
- Increased cardiac damage during a heart attack [10]

 ON THE HORIZON

New treatments for traumatic shock are in development. Currently, opioid receptor antagonists, such as naloxone and naltrexone, are used to reverse traumatic shock. These drugs antagonize opioid receptors in a nonselective way, including mu receptors. When administered, pain levels soar. Drugs currently in development that selectively antagonize delta and kappa opioid receptors likely will treat shock more effectively without drastically increasing the pain experienced by patients with traumatic shock [7].

- Tachycardia, hypertension, increased myocardial demand, hypercoagulation
- Disturbed sleep
- Hormonal disturbances (ACTH, cortisol, catecholamines, and insulin) [11–13]
- Hastened cancer metastasis [14]
- Infection or impaired healing [15]
- Shallow breathing with impaired lung clearing [16]
- Atelectasis and nosocomial pneumonia [8, 16]
- Incurable chronic pain syndromes [17–21]

Pain also prevents people from being active. This leads to longer hospital stays and delayed recovery. Specific results of immobility in hospitalized patients include:

- Increased risk of thromboembolism
- Muscle spasms, atrophy, and limited range of motion
- Bone demineralization
- Increased risk of infection
- Increased risk of impaired skin integrity
- Cardiopulmonary deconditioning

Given these harms associated with unrelieved pain, nurses are reminded of their ethical duty to provide prompt, effective relief as is detailed in Chapter 1.

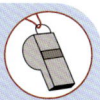

COACH CONSULT

At any age, severe pain creates changes in physiology throughout the body, including changing the structure and function of nerves. Neonates are vulnerable to the long-term effects of severe and repeated pain. The effect on feeding, sleeping, and self-regulation is transient, but permanent damage can result from intraventricular hemorrhage linked to the stress of severe pain. Attention deficit and learning disorders also have been linked to neonatal pain [22]. Pain is believed to prevent the natural pruning back of excess nerves and synapses in the neonatal brain. This altered brain architecture can increase sensitivity to stimuli, including the creation of a sustained hypersensitivity to pain.

Pathological Pain

Normally, nociceptors are quiet, becoming active only in response to intense, potentially harmful stimuli. Damaged tissue amplifies, spreads, and prolongs the activity of these nerves. Most often, pain enhancers— or active nociceptors—are temporary and resolve when damaged tissues heal. Usually, the signals that facilitate and inhibit pain are in balance, so that individuals are neither hypersensitive nor insensitive to pain for any length of time. In patients with painful degenerative conditions, ongoing inflammation, or nerve damage, this balance can become upset and transform pain from a symptom into a chronic, degenerative, and incurable disorder.

Acute pain represents a biologically useful warning mechanism and can be likened to an alarm clock. An irritating signal tells the body to get moving and stop the annoyance. Once the alarm serves its purpose, it turns off until needed again. Chronic neuropathic pain can be likened to a broken alarm clock. It serves no useful purpose, getting louder and more annoying over time, with no means to shut it off.

Chronic pain produces pathological changes in the nerves, and an alteration in nerve function. If intense pain persists for more than a couple of hours, inflammatory or neuropathic changes create additional pain-signaling problems [23, 24]. Structural changes in the nerves include:

- Increase or decrease of the number of specific receptors and ion channel types
- Growth of new types of receptors and ion channels
- Sprouts of new axons and dendrites (see Fig. 3–5)
- New synaptic connections
- Reorganization of dorsal horn and pain-processing centers of brain

Although these structural and functional changes in the nervous system may be reversible if pain is controlled in the first hours or days; when they persist for weeks or months these changes are believed to be irreversible. This accounts for the persistence of pain long after the original tissue damage has healed.

Changes in nerve functioning that increase sensitivity to stimuli and allow pain transmission to be sustained over time include:

- Change in resting membrane potential and activation threshold
- Abnormal forms of signal transduction
  - Cross talk between nerves
  - Spontaneous ectopic nerve firing
- Change in action potentials when nerves are stimulated
  - Increase in nerve-firing rate
  - Amplification of signal strength
  - Long-term potentiation prolongs the nerve's activity
- Change in type and intensity of stimulus needed to generate a response

Nerve Structural Changes

The brain is not a hardwired, fixed structure with stable and predictable response patterns [22]. From the moment of birth, the brain rapidly adapts to changing internal and external environments. A single, strong stimulus or repeated weak stimuli create a memory in the brain that

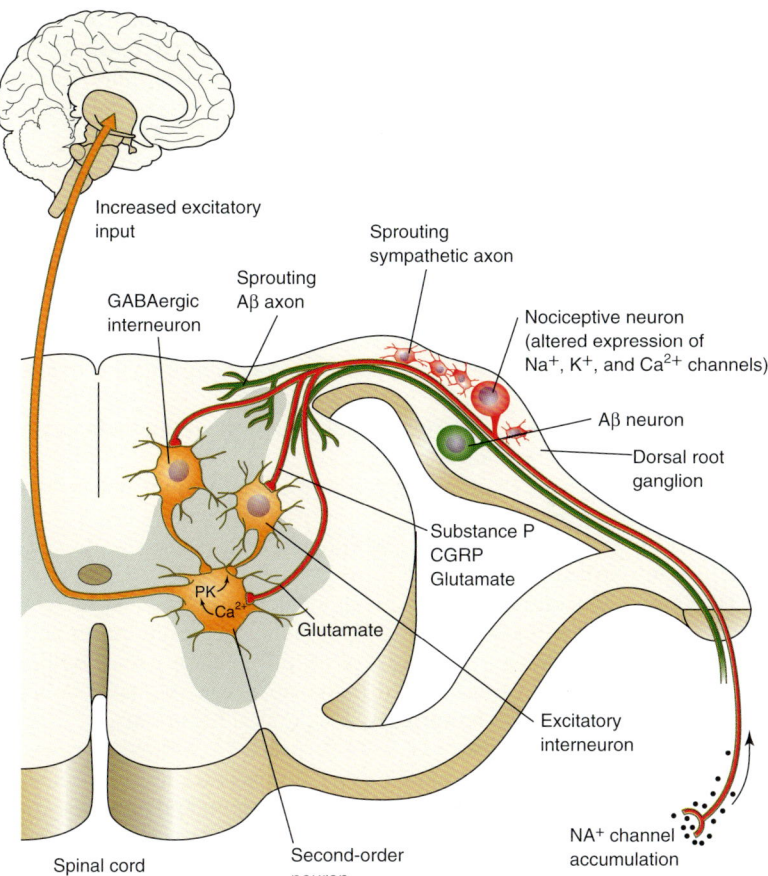

FIGURE 3-5: Neuropathic changes contributing to chronic pain: key alterations in nerves occur in pathological pain states. Transformations involve a change in density of specific receptors and ion channel types, sprouts of new axons and dendrites, including abnormal tangles between pain fibers, sympathetic nerves and touch (Aβ) fibers.

increases reactivity (sensitivity) to future stimuli. This sensitization begins because synapses, receptors, and ion channels have become more efficient, having had more "practice." They have become more efficient at initiating and transmitting warning signals to the brain. This process of transmission becomes maladaptive, however, when alerts are generated and sent either in error or in the absence of danger [24].

Ion Channel and Receptor Changes

Among the smallest structures to change are the specific ion channels and their receptors. Positively charged ions create the "spark" generating nerve impulses. Factors that increase the intracellular concentration of positively charged ions facilitate abnormal nerve activity. Those changes associated with pathological pain include:

- Na^+ channels multiply in damaged nerves, neuromas, and dorsal root ganglia
- Vanilloid receptors multiply on peripheral pain fiber, increasing their Ca^{++} permeability
- Calming K^+ ion channels, which move positive ions out of nerves become sparse and less active
- Chloride channels allow negatively charged ions to escape rather than permeate nerves

The higher concentration of positively charged ions, yields changes in density, distribution, and action of ion channels. As a result, nerve activation thresholds are lower, requiring less stimuli to elicit pain. Combined with shortened nerve resting times, this change causes spontaneous activity, even in the absence of stimuli and accelerated firing rates.

Glutamate-NMDA Activation

When nerves are sensitized to pain, Ca^{++} channels become more efficient. The rise of presynaptic Ca^{++} stimulates prostaglandin and excitatory neurotransmitter (glutamate) release. This release initiates a feed-forward mechanism that produces the following problematic sequence of events:

1. Active Ca^{++} channels increase production and release of glutamate
2. Excitatory glutamate augments NMDA receptors
3. Glutamate interacts with NMDA receptors, removing a magnesium block
4. Excitatory calcium floods the cells, stimulating glutamate production and release

This glutamate-NMDA activation causes an excitatory state by lowering postsynaptic activation thresholds, resulting in spontaneous nerve activity and a hyperalgesic state. Eventually, this glutamate-NMDA-Ca^{++} interaction can produce a neurotoxic state that causes degeneration and death of dorsal horn neurons [25, 26]. This neuron death creates a void that is filled by new sprouts that are highly sensitive to pain, generating the hypersensitivity and allodynia often seen with pathological pain.

Hyperalgesia

Hyperalgesia is a state of pain amplification. In addition to the CNS buildup of excitatory neurotransmitters and positively charged ions, more AMPA* receptors are produced. These receptors interact with NMDA sites to stimulate C-fiber windup, sodium permeability, and long-term potentiation. This windup amplifies pain intensity while long-term potentiation changes the dorsal horn and brain in a way that produces prolonged nerve firing that extends pain duration.

While this upsurge in excitatory factors takes place, there is a simultaneous decline of inhibitory factors [3]. Spinal inhibitory interneurons are usually abundant in the superficial dorsal horn. These interneurons provide presynaptic inhibition by modulating the activity of GABA and glycine. Peripheral nerve injury decreases GABA receptors in the dorsal horn, which in turn reduces both presynaptic and postsynaptic inhibition.

Pathological (neuropathic) pain states often do not respond fully to opioids. In part, this may result from the substantial reduction in CNS opioid receptors [2, 22]. Opioid receptors become internalized through a process of endocytosis, so they are not available on the cell membrane to respond to available opioids. Dynorphin, an opioid receptor agonist, also initiates glutamate release, contributing to dorsal horn excitability. In the absence of normal opioid receptors, dynorphin can take on a purely excitatory function.

 ON THE HORIZON

When opioids fail to provide more than partial temporary relief of neuropathic pain, adjuvant medications are used to oppose nervous system changes that contribute to abnormal pain processing. Antidepressants used for pain block the reuptake of both noradrenaline and serotonin, thereby enhancing descending inhibition. Tricyclic antidepressants also produce some NMDA-receptor antagonism and sodium-channel blockade. Anticonvulsant drugs, such as gabapentin, stabilize the nerves by blocking calcium channels. Lidocaine and mexiletine block Na^+ channels, while capsaicin depletes stores of substance P.

---

*AMPA receptors (made up of alpha-amino-3-hydroxy-5-methyl-4-isoxazolepropionic acid), similar to NMDA receptors, are activated by the excitatory amino acid, glutamate.

Nerve Growth and Reorganization

Neuroplastic changes take place peripherally and centrally, which are capable to amplifying and prolonging pain. These nerve reorganization processes can include:

- Activation of silent nociceptors
- Nerve growth
- Sprouting of abnormal sympathetic nerve components
- Cross talk between nerves
- Reorganization of the brain
- Activation of immune cells

Activation of Silent Nociceptors

Inflammation and sensitization of peripheral nerves wakes up silent nociceptors, which become additional vehicles capable of signaling, amplifying, and spreading pain [27]. In skin, musculoskeletal, and visceral tissue, an estimated one-third of all C-fibers and one-half of A-delta fibers are normally insensitive, even to strong manipulation by mechanical stimuli. Once awakened, however, these silent nociceptors respond to a range of mechanical, chemical, and thermal stimuli. Normally, these nociceptors return to a sleeping state when inflammation subsides. In pathological states, however, they remain active and hypersensitive [23].

Nerve Growth

Nerve growth factor (NGF) is required for the long-term growth, survival, and differentiation of nerve cells. NGF can regulate the sensitivity of sensory nerves and mediate processes of inflammation that can amplify pain. This occurs in peripheral and central nerves. Peripherally, after nerve injury, distal nerve segments initially die back, followed by sprouting of new axons and receptors [28]. The resultant neuroma, a chaotic tangle of overgrown nerve endings, can be a source of long-term pain when:

- Growth cone sprouts fail to reach the original target of the damaged nerve
- Tangled nerve tissue overproduces Na^+ channels that have lower transduction thresholds (chemical and mechanical sensitivity) than the original nerve
- Cross talk develops when adjacent nerve activity triggers an errant pain signal

Problematic growth of central nerves in response to elevated NGF includes:

- Growth of new axons, dendrites, synapses, receptors, and ion channels

- Sprouting nerve growths can develop self-stimulating reverberating loops
- Increased sensitivity to stimuli types and lowered thresholds for firing action potentials
- Change in the type and amount of neurotransmitters produced and released
- Creation of abnormal linkages between pain fibers and other sensory or sympathetic nerves

NGF has an important role in the development of pathological pain states.

Sprouting of Abnormal Sympathetic Nerve Components

Injured sensory nerves release NGF that stimulates the growth of alpha-adrenergic receptors and postganglionic sympathetic sprouts on peripheral nerves [23]. Nerve injury also causes sprouting of sympathetic fibers that invade and form basketlike structures around the dorsal root ganglion. These structures function as synapses that provide an additional source of errant ectopic discharges perceived as pain [28]. These sprouts release noradrenaline, which can directly activate sleeping nociceptors. Indirectly, sympathetic and sensory nerves engage in cross talk, allowing the stimulation of normally insensate sympathetic nerve fibers to activate adjacent pain-signaling nerves. These sympathetic sprouts are coupled with nociceptors and acquire the capacity to evoke pain, especially during times of stress.

Cross Talk

Cross talk occurs deep in the spine, where low-threshold touch fibers stimulate normally high-threshold pain fibers located more superficially in the spine. Hair blowing in the breeze (a low-threshold stimulus) can elicit pain signals that usually require a much higher-intensity stimulus (e.g., a forceful slap) to respond. Normal, intact nerves, transmit impulses through well-insulated channels. When the integrity of these channels is disrupted by illness or injury, cross talk (also termed *ephaptic transmission*) occurs between adjacent nerve fibers [3]. A-beta fibers (signaling light touch) sprout into superficial dorsal spine regions where pain signals are transmitted [3, 28]. This synaptic reorganization produces cross talk between these nerves, resulting in light touch being perceived as pain (mechanical allodynia).

Reorganization of the Brain

Neuroplastic (structural and functional) changes in the brain disrupt the normal processes responsible for the perception, understanding of, and responses to pain. After peripheral nerve injury, cell death occurs in the brain, resulting in cortical and subcortical reorganization [5, 29]. The void left by dead brain cells is "filled in" by the growth of new sprouts from adjacent nerve cells. After substantial injury, such as an amputation, subsequent restructuring (dying back and filling in) may encompass large areas of the sensory-motor cortex. This can include:

- Memory traces from earlier experiences with pain
- Heightened excitability from central sensitization
- Spontaneous nerve firing, with or without peripheral stimulation
- Impaired ability to discriminate the type and location of pain
- The sensation of abnormal position sense or movement of the amputated body part

In chronic pain states, the dorsal horn, thalamus, prefrontal cortex, and other areas of the brain begin to degenerate. The result of degeneration is in metabolic change, cell death, and brain atrophy or loss of gray matter. Loss of gray matter has been linked directly to perception of pain intensity and duration. For those with chronic pain, loss of brain tissue continues at a rate of 1.5 cm³ per year above that associated with normal aging [5, 27]. Pain relief does increase thalamic activity, but the degree to which cerebral atrophy and other degenerative brain changes are reversible remains unclear.

Activation of Immune Cells

Immune cells, mast cells, and macrophages flood damaged or hyperactive areas of the CNS. Immune cells are typically a protective mechanism but in this situation they can go awry. Some act to increase sensitivity to pain, specifically:

- Astrocytes increase secretion and slow the reuptake of the excitatory amino acid glutamate
- Glial cells secrete glutamate and inflammation-provoking prostaglandins

Of these changes in the immune system, the activation and multiplication of glial cells may be more important. Thousands of glial cells, acting as CNS macrophages, engulf damaged or hyperactive neurons. Upon

---

 NURSE-TO-NURSE TIP

Using high-dose opioids following nerve damage may paradoxically amplify pain. Dynorphin, glutamate, and activation of NMDA receptors create a neurotoxic buildup of calcium and excitatory amino acids. Dark neurons form, malfunction, die, and are replaced with excitatory cells, resulting in hyperalgesia or allodynia. When pain escalates or spreads chronic for conditions previously controlled with opioids, consider opioid-induced hyperalgesia as a possible etiology. Dose reduction or switching medications may be needed to treat this form of worsening pain.

---

engulfment, the glia release inflammation-producing substances, such as substance P, bradykinin, and prostaglandins that in turn amplify pain [3, 15]. Some people are believed to have a genetic condition whereby they lack the ability to terminate this glial assault, which may account for some disease states (e.g., fibromyalgia) or familial vulnerability to chronic pain.

Altered Perception of Pain

Scientists are just beginning to develop the tools and models needed to understand the complex mechanisms of pain perception in patients with pathological and chronic pain. Patients with chronic pain have a higher level of activity in the prefrontal cortex and a lower level of activity in the thalamus than patients with acute, normal responses to pain [5, 30]. When chronic pain—as opposed to normal pain—is relieved, there is a spike in thalamic activity. The limbic regions of the brain (i.e., ACC, insula, amygdale, and frontal cortex) also play an important role in the perception, recall, and unpleasantness of abnormal pain states, such as allodynia [31]. These physiological differences correspond with the clinical observation that those with chronic pain have a heightened awareness of affective and cognitive aspects of pain and dulled sensory-discriminative perceptions of it.

 NURSE-TO-NURSE TIP

Although it may be tempting to dismiss a patient's report of pain in situations where the underlying mechanism cannot be explained, labeling pain as "all in the head" undermines the development of a therapeutic relationship. Rather than assuming a psychogenic cause, this type of pain is more accurately described as idiopathic, or of unknown cause. Most of the pathological mechanisms described in this chapter escape detection by diagnostic tests. Knowing that these pathological changes can be driven by untreated pain should compel the nurse to seek optimal and expedient pain control whether or not the pain's origin is understood.

4 Pain Assessment

Assessment

CHAPTER 4

Pain Assessment

A skilled assessment lays the groundwork for optimal pain management. When properly done, it will guide interventions and provide the baseline for comparison to evaluate treatment. Timely, skilled pain reassessments are needed to determine the safety, and efficacy of interventions, and to refine the treatment plan based on individual needs and responses.

In some patients, a skilled pain assessment is as straightforward as asking a few simple questions; but, for others, more advanced assessment techniques are required. For all patients numerous factors can affect their perception of, and reaction to pain. These include:

- Personal, ethnic, and cultural values
- Emotional traits
- Personality
- Developmental stage
- Previous pain experiences

Additionally, the following situational factors contribute to the current perception of and behavioral response to pain:

- Immediate physical and social environment
- Current affect (e.g., anxiety, fear, depression)
- Motivation and meaning of pain (e.g., perceived interference with planned activities, threat of serious consequences)

Nurses should realize that they can influence many of these factors, and can inadvertently amplify or intentionally dampen the physical and emotional intensity of the experience [1].

NURSE-TO-NURSE TIP

Historically, the training and practice settings of many nurses have been dominated by a culture that values stoicism; this has lead to the view that tolerance of pain is a sign of strength. Patients who are more expressive about their pain and emotions may be labeled as "weak," "demanding," or "whimps" with subtle comments, body language, or professional actions capable of reinforcing or extinguishing those behaviors. Studies examining why patients suffer in silence with uncontrolled pain consistently reveal that the majority of patients do not want to be labeled as complainers [2, 3]. "Labeling" a patient, or questioning the validity of their expressions about pain, can actually worsen pain and suffering. It is most helpful to accept the expression of pain as a person's way of communicating an unmet need, and focus nursing time on meeting identified needs in an effective, expedient way.

Standards of Pain Assessment

According to The Joint Commission standards for pain assessment [4]:
- All patients will be asked whether they have pain
- Patients will be informed of their right to have pain assessed and managed
- Patients will be told about how pain is assessed and managed
- When pain is present, a detailed assessment will be done in accordance with the patient's:
  - Age
  - Condition
  - Ability to understand
- A reassessment of pain is done based on the organization's specified criteria
- All nurses, doctors, and professionals dealing with pain must be trained to do so

These and other standards translate into a requirement that all patients need to be screened for the presence of pain:
- On admission
- When transferred from one facility (or unit) to another
- After a procedure requiring strong sedative or anesthetic drugs to be used

Once pain is determined to be present, a thorough assessment of pain must be performed by professionals who also have a duty to treat or refer the patient for pain treatment. Subsequent reassessment of pain is required following the intervention [4]. This section will cover:

- Brief screening for pain and distress
- Systematic approach to assessing and reassessing pain
- Modified approaches to assessing pain in specific patient populations

Brief Screening for Pain

Given that many people with mild or moderate pain will not talk about their pain unless asked about it, screening for the presence of pain must be done before the pain escalates to intolerable levels. Subtle differences in the wording and tone of screening questions affect the patient's willingess to disclose useful clinical information about his or her pain. Astute nurses analyze the words used by patients to gain insights to their underlying needs (see Table 4–1).

Having a clear rating scale also is needed once the presence of pain is established. A scale of "1 to 10" is confusing because "1" has no meaning. Using zero as the lowest point on the scale (e.g., "0 to 10") is better understood, because "no pain" is instantly recognizable. If the patient is having a difficult time rating the pain on a numeric scale, use some other method (e.g., verbal description) that can be translated by the nurse into a number (see Fig. 4–1).

It also is essential that nurses listen to and accept the patient's perceptions of pain as reported. Accepting the person's report of discomfort is central to establishing the sense of trust needed to develop and sustain a therapeutic relationship. If the patient states he or she has no discomfort,

COACH CONSULT

The abbreviation "no c/o" may be documented in progress notes. Officially, that abbreviation means "no complaints offered." Sometimes this is used to incorrectly imply that, because the patient did not complain, no pain was experienced. This abbreviation tends to be used in lieu of direct assessment. Similarly, the abbreviation "WNL" is sometimes used to suggest "within normal limits," when really the assessment was not done properly, suggesting that WNL may really mean "we never looked." Instead, the nurse must ask the patient about his or her pain and, if none, document "denies pain."

 WHY IS WORDING IMPORTANT?

Asking about "discomforts" generally will yield more information than asking first about "pain." Words, such as "bad" or "complain" also have emotional or sociocultural meanings attached that make some patients reluctant to report their discomforts, thus these terms should be avoided.

Table 4–1 **Common Words Describing Pain and Distress**		
EMOTIONAL DISTRESS	NEUROPATHIC PAIN	NOCICEPTIVE PAIN
Frightening	Burning	Tender
Punishing	Flashing	Sharp, cutting
Vicious	Shooting	Dull
Annoying	Stabbing	Cramping
Nagging	Tingling	Squeezing
Unbearable	Prickling	Throbbing

the nurse can record no pain and further screenings or reassessments of pain are done at intervals determined by institutional policy. If the patient reports the presence of pain, the nurse should perform a more comprehensive pain assessment. Some institutions permit both licensed and unlicensed personnel to screen for pain, however, the comprehensive assessment is conducted by a trained professional.

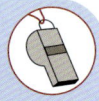

COACH CONSULT

Avoid subtle mistakes when screening for pain. Do not ask: "Do you have any complaints of pain?" Patients are reluctant to discuss pain because they do not want to complain. It is better to ask, "Are you having any pain or discomfort?"

The nurse and patient often sidestep discussions about the patient's emotional state until it escalates to the level of severe distress. Given that pain is universally an unpleasant experience, letting the patient know that pain is always a physical *and* emotional experience may facilitate patient disclosure. Because unpleasant emotions are capable of amplifying and prolonging the physical sensations of pain, assessing distress becomes pertinent to the evaluation and treatment of pain.

To screen for both the sensory and emotional components of pain, the nurse can:
- Inform patients that physical and emotional discomforts are routinely evaluated
- Ask the patient to describe the physical sensation that is bothering him or her the most
  - With multiple areas of pain, focus on the area of the worst pain first
  - Seek descriptions of the sensation (e.g., sharp, aching, shooting, burning)

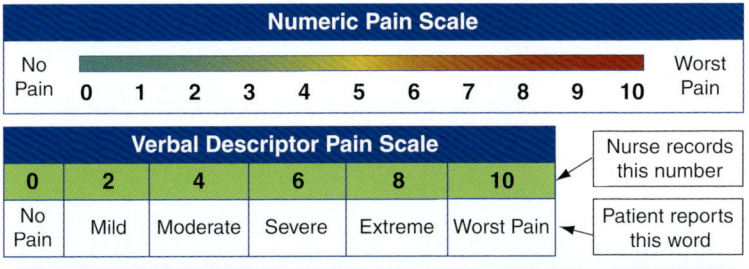

Numeric Pain Scale

| No Pain | 0 | 1 | 2 | 3 | 4 | 5 | 6 | 7 | 8 | 9 | 10 | Worst Pain |

Verbal Descriptor Pain Scale

0	2	4	6	8	10	
No Pain	Mild	Moderate	Severe	Extreme	Worst Pain	

Nurse records this number

Patient reports this word

Functional Pain Scale*

0	2	4	6	8	10
No Pain	Activities unaffected	Prevents some active activities	Prevents all active, (not passive) activities	Prevents all passive activities	Incapacitated, unable to even speak due to pain

Tolerable .... **Intolerable**

Active activities: usual activities or those requiring effort (turning, walking, etc.)
Passive activities: talking on phone watching TV, reading

*Scale modified slightly to adhere to policy of using a 0–10 scale

Checklist for Nonverbal Pain Indicators	When moves	At rest	Total
Vocal Expressions: Moans, groans, grunts, cries, sighs, says "ouch/hurt"			
Facial Expression: Wince, grimace, furrowed brow, tight lips/jaw			
Bracing: Clutches; holds side rails, bed, table, or area of pain			
Restlessness: Shifts position, hand movements, unable to keep still			
Rubbing: Touching, holding, rubbing, or massaging affected area			
		TOTAL SCORE:	

FIGURE 4–1: Sample MPAR used at Massachusetts General Hospital with first-line scale (Numeric Pain Scale) and methods to obtain a 0–10 score for patients unable to provide a number.

- To promote understanding the scale, ask the patient if he or she would recognize "0"—a state of no pain (or no aching) and "10" the worst pain (aching) imaginable
  - Patient then rates sensation intensity "right now" between those points
- Have patient describe the most bothersome current emotion (e.g., worried, mad, afraid)
- Define the rating scale anchors (e.g., "0" not at all mad; "10" as mad as possible)
  - Patient rates emotional intensity "right now" between those points

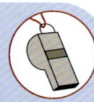

COACH CONSULT

Document the patient's description of his or her pain verbatim. Pain is a subjective experience, often defined as "whatever the person says it is" [5]. A change in the description of the pain, over time or in response to treatment, is clinically important. Record the description of the pain using the patient's words rather than the nurse's.

Patients who describe their pain in emotional terms, such as killing, annoying, frightening, excruciating, or unbearable, should be encouraged to validate the emotions they are experiencing and to rate the emotional intensity on a 0-to-10 scale. After completing the emotional rating, have the patient try to describe the physical sensation he or she is experiencing and then rate it on a 0-to-10 scale. Review Table 4–1 for common words used to describe pain and distress.

Systematic Approach to Assessing and Reassessing Pain

Given the multidimensional (e.g., biopsychosocial) nature of pain, a systematic approach is needed to ensure accuracy and completeness of the evaluation. Gender, culture, social interactions, and prior personal pain experiences shape the individual's perception of his or her pain and ability to share details with the nurse. In general, women are better able to perceive and discriminate different types of pain, while men are more reluctant to talk about their pain or seek professional treatment [6]. In some cultures, pain expression is associated with a punishment for sins, and its expression may result in shame. Subtle behavioral changes may be the only clue a nurse has that pain is problematic. The nurse who communicates in a calm, nonjudgmental, and culturally aware manner can help the patient overcome reluctance to discuss discomforts [7]. Although it begins with a simple question, a comprehensive pain assessment is a systematic and ongoing process involving the patient, family, and other health-care providers [8].

Obtaining the Patient's Self-Report of Pain

The patient's verbal report of pain is considered the most accurate measurement available. The subjective account of one's experience, combined with clinical data and psychosocial factors, such as related thoughts, feelings, and actions, comprise a comprehensive pain assessment. Several acronyms have been used to help guide nurses through the interview portion of the pain assessment.

The WILDA Pain Assessment Guide simplifies the pain assessment process for nurses by focusing on five key components [9] they need to ask about pain, including:

- **W**ords (describe the discomfort, such as sharp, stabbing, or aching)
- **I**ntensity (severity of pain)
- **L**ocation (body parts that are uncomfortable)
- **D**uration (pattern of pain over time)
- **A**ggravating and **A**lleviating factors (what makes pain better and what makes it worse)

Words

The words patients use to describe their pain helps the nurse consider the underlying treatable cause of pain that needs to be addressed. When used during the recovery or postoperative phase, it can help nurses distinguish between expected and unanticipated pains. For example, if Ms. Forbes was recovering from abdominal surgery, descriptions of her discomfort may be sharp or achy to describe the incisional pain she is likely to experience. However, if Ms. Forbes described a severe pressure, throbbing, or cramping kind of pain, this may represent a common complication, such as an ileus, or serious internal bleeding; both of which warrant different types of evaluation and treatment. Words can help differentiate the kind of pain described by a patient: pain related to the primary condition, a complication, or some other coincidental problem that needs a separate evaluation and treatment

Intensity

Using a number to represent the intensity of pain can facilitate communication and continuity of care [10]. To accomplish this, the number must have meaning to the patients and professionals involved. Having the emergency room using a 0-to-100 pain-rating scale while the intensive care unit uses a 1-to-6 scale and the general care units use a 0-to-10 scale is confusing, so most organizations adopt a 0 (no pain)-to-10 (worst pain) scale as the standard metric for pain intensity. The inclusion of word modifiers on the scale can assist some patients who find it difficult to apply a number level to their pain (see Fig. 4–1).

For example, after ruling out "0" and "10" (neither no pain nor the worst possible pain), a nurse can ask the patient if the pain intensity is mild, moderate, severe, or extreme in nature, and record the number 2, 4, 6, or 8 respectively. The scoring range is such that if the patient reports pain is between mild and moderate, the nurse can record a "3" as his or her pain intensity score.

Another way to explain the intensity of pain for patients having trouble understanding the numeric rating scale is to determine the extent of pain awareness and degree to which it interferes with functioning [11]. The following descriptions use the 0-to-10 scale by considering the tolerance of certain activities:

- Patients who deny the presence of pain are scored "0"
- A "2" can be ignored without diminishing active (usual or desirable) activities
- A "4" can be tolerated, but some active activities are avoided due to pain
- A "6" is intolerable and interferes with all active activities, but the patient can still do passive activities, such as watch TV, talk on the phone, or read a book
- An "8" interferes with all active and passive activities
- A "10" is the worst possible pain. It is intense and incapacitating allowing for no active or passive activities, rendering the person unable to communicate about anything besides pain

Location

Noting the location of pain is crucial, not only during the initial assessment, but also throughout the course of treatment. In the case of Ms. Forbes described above, a severe abdominal pain in the area of her surgery would be less alarming than if she had a new onset of severe chest pain, headache, or leg pains, which could signal serious postoperative complications.

Although pain typically presents in the area of the body where the problem exists, some pains present in different locations or may radiate from one part of the body to another. For example, a gallbladder attack may present as right shoulder (subscapular) pain; or a myofascial trigger point can hurt in the shoulder and send pain down the arm on the involved side. In many patients, especially those with chronic pain, there may be more than one site of pain. Each site must be assessed separately to determine type of pain and potential treatment.

Duration

Evaluating the duration, detailing the pattern of pain over time is important. The nurse gathers information about the circumstances and time the pain began; how it has changed since then; how long the pain lasts; whether it recurs and, if so, the timing of intervals with and without pain; and when the pain last occurred. Attention to the pattern of pain helps the nurse anticipate and meet the needs of the patient, and recognize patterns of grave concern.

Aggravating and Alleviating Factors

Evaluating the aggravating and alleviating factors affecting pain intensity can help refine the diagnosis, care plan, and treatment strategy. For example, a patient with peptic ulcer disease who describes whether the intake of food worsens or relieves pain can help distinguish an ulcer in the stomach from one in the duodenum [12]. Awareness of the time it takes analgesics to alleviate pain and the time of scheduled painful therapeutic exercises, helps the nurse provide preemptive analgesia so pain will be lower at times of therapy to maximize patient involvement. In addition to identifying pain triggers that can be avoided or altered, factors that reduce pain can be combined, such as topical heat while assuming a position of comfort plus distracting attention, during episodes of pain (or analgesic gaps) to provide additive relief.

> **ALERT** ❗
>
> Be alert for abrupt changes in pain intensity. For example, the abrupt cessation of acute abdominal pain, after a period of steadily intensifying pain, may indicate that an inflamed appendix has ruptured.

Asking About Other Symptoms and the Effect of Pain

Beyond inquiring about pain using the WILDA method, two other aspects need to be explored (see Table 4–2) to complete the assessment, including:

1. Ask about other symptoms besides pain that bother the patient
2. Note the effect of pain on daily activities, and on physical, mental, and social well-being.

Other concurrent symptoms are important to consider while assessing and treating pain.

Nausea often is experienced with pain arising from a visceral origin (e.g., gastritis). It may also be a side effect of analgesics or a symptom of opioid withdrawal. With a post-traumatic headache, the presence of nausea or vomiting can signal a dangerous rise in intracranial pressure. Diaphoresis, dyspnea, or excessive fatigue similarly can indicate a more serious cause of chest pain and help distinguish a heart attack from heartburn (see Table 4–2).

The effect of pain on usual sleep and activity patterns also provides useful information. Acute pain severe enough to interfere with sleep is typically more serious than pain that does not awaken. Sleep interruption

Table 4–2 Other Symptoms and the Effect of Pain to Evaluate	
OTHER SYMPTOMS*	EFFECTS OF PAIN
Fever, fatigue, weight loss	Sleep
Diaphoresis, dyspnea, or palpitations	Appetite
Circulation, sensation, or motor changes	Usual physical activities and recreation
Changes in vision and/or hearing	Interpersonal relations
Nausea, vomiting and/or anorexia	Role functioning (e.g., home, family, and work)
Urine or stool pattern changes	Financial
Change in cognition or level of consciousness	Mood

*These other symptoms are important to note in patients with pain as they may aid in the diagnosis and treatment of potentially serious underlying problems.

or excessive sleep with chronic pain may signal the development of depression. Evaluating the effect pain has on daily living activities, such as eating, walking, working, driving, and social or recreational activities, provides important information needed to effectively treat pain and guide rehabilitation efforts. Some patients are distraught by their inability to fulfill caretaker responsibilities. This anxiety can amplify the sensation and emotional distress until assistance is in place to meet the need of others who rely on them. Therefore, it is important to determine the effect pain has on roles, responsibilities and the ability to participate in meaningful activities. When severe pain persists for a year or longer, depression is pervasive, which further intensifies pain and its psychosocial affect.

COACH CONSULT

Did you remember to ask about all parts of pain?
• Words
• Intensity
• Location
• Duration
• Aggravating and alleviating factors
• Other symptoms
• Effects on physical, mental, and social activities

Observing the Patient's Physiological and Behavioral Signs of Pain

Physiological and behavioral signs of pain are poor indicators of pain, so they should not be used to discredit or override the patient's self-report of pain. Paying attention to these signs however, can provide additional useful information to complement the verbal report of discomforts. For patients who cannot communicate verbally, general physiological and behavioral signs, such as tachycardia and grimacing, respectively, provide information about pain to compensate for the lack of information about the patients' perceptions of discomfort.

Physiologic Indicators of Pain

Physiologic responses vary with the origin and duration of the pain. The onset of acute pain stimulates the sympathetic nervous system, resulting in:

- Increased blood pressure (> 10% to 20% increase)
- Increased pulse rate
- Rapid, shallow respirations
- Pallor
- Diaphoresis
- Pupil dilation

The body does not sustain the increased sympathetic function over a prolonged period of time and, therefore, the sympathetic nervous system adapts, making the physiologic responses less evident or even absent [13]. Physiologic responses are more likely to be absent in people with chronic pain because of autonomic nervous system adaptation that usually takes place minutes after the onset of pain. Measures of physiologic responses, such as pulse and blood pressure, are poor indicators of the presence, absence, or severity of pain and should be used only when self-report is not possible.

Behavioral Indicators of Pain

Patients who are very young, aphasic, confused, or disoriented may not be able to verbalize their discomforts, making nonverbal behavior their only means of communicating pain. There are wide variations in nonverbal responses to pain. Facial expression is often the first indication of pain [13], and it may be the only one. Common behavioral indicators of pain are:

- Clenched teeth, tightly shut (or open, somber) eyes, or grimacing
- Vocalizations, such as moaning, groaning, crying, or screaming
- Immobilization, guarding, holding, or rubbing the hurt body part
- Stiff or awkward movements (e.g., limping, fetal position, or tightly gripping side rails, etc.)

Purposeless body movements, such as tossing and turning in bed or flailing extremities, also can indicate pain. Involuntary or purposeful movements, such as a reflexive jerking away from a needle inserted through the skin or striking at someone who would try, can indicate pain. An adult may be able to control this reflex; a child may be unable or unwilling to do so. Rhythmic body movements or rubbing may indicate pain. An adult or child may assume a fetal position and rock back and forth

ALERT !

It is important to note that behavioral responses often can be controlled, so their presence or absence may not be very revealing and should be substantiated with another means of assessment (e.g., self-report or surrogate report) when possible.

when experiencing abdominal pain. During labor a woman may massage her abdomen rhythmically with her hands.

Physical Assessment of a Patient with Pain

The patient interview is followed by a careful examination of the painful area to reveal treatable causes of the pain, such as foreign bodies or structural anomalies [13]. Gentle palpation of the painful area will help identify warmth (related to inflammation), or abnormal pain sensitivity (hypersensitivity or allodynia) that demands further evaluation to rule out serious complications. In addition to examining and palpating the area of pain, nurses assess pertinent bodily systems that may be contributing to the pain [13]. Conducting an assessment of the circulatory, neurological, and musculoskeletal systems is prudent for extremity pain; a gastrointestinal and genitourinary system assessment is warranted for abdominal pain; a cardiopulmonary assessment is needed for chest pain.

Reassessment of Pain

Reassessments of the intensity and quality of pain and responses to treatments are required following any procedure, change in condition, or other transition (i.e., transfer, discharge) in care (see Fig. 4–2). Patient responses to interventions will vary; therefore reassessments are tailored to clinical factors and individual goals [14]. Pain reduction is often quantified on a numeric scale or a percent the pain is reduced after an intervention. Typically, a 50% reduction in acute pain and a 30% reduction in chronic pain are considered the benchmark of clinical success.

🗨 NURSE-TO-NURSE TIP

For non-English speaking patients, use tools in their native language and an interpreter to aid in assessments. Recognize, however, that the interpreter's gender, perceptions, and attitudes may influence the quantity and quality of information conveyed. Given that disclosing pain to a family member or to a person of the opposite sex may be culturally inappropriate, trained interpreters should be used instead of family members. Trained interpreters can serve as valuable "cultural brokers" who facilitate communication and understanding of the social and cultural context of their experience.

Massachusetts General Hospital Pain Assessment & Reassessment (M-PAR©) Procedure

Pain Assessment:

All patients are screened for the presence of pain on admission, transfer and after procedures. When pain is present, more details need to be evaluated in addition to intensity, such as: sensation descriptors, location, pattern (constant, intermittent), factors that intensify or alleviate pain and effects on activity or bio-psycho-social functioning. The acronym, **WILDA**, can be used to guide this expanded assessment.

W	**Words** describing pain
I	**Intensity** (severity on 0-10 scale)
L	**Location** (body part affected)
D	**Duration** (change since starting)
A	**Aggravating/Alleviating** factors

Pain Reassessment:

Timely, skilled reassessment of pain is needed to determine the safety and efficacy of intervention, as well as individualize treatment plans based response. Reassessments of the intensity, quality and responses to treatments are required following the administration of any analgesic. Reassessments are timed to coincide with anticipated effects of the analgesic (e.g. within 1 hour after prn dose) and every 4 hours for patients with scheduled analgesics, continuous, PCA or epidural infusions. Three essential components of reassessments are summarized as the **3-A's; Activity, Adverse effects, and Analgesia.**

1) **A**ctivity: Note level of improvement due to reduced interference from pain, and any safety issues related to risk of injury due to the effects of the medicine.

2) **A**dverse effects: Note any signs of side effects, toxicity, technology-related complications or aberrant behaviors. Specifically, note sedation, respiratory depression or abdominal pain.

3) **A**nalgesia: this can be done in 1 of 3 ways
   a) Rate the pain intensity on the same scale before and after the intervention –or-
   b) Ask the patient to estimate a percent reduction in the pain intensity – or-
   c) Ask for a description of the amount of relief, (some relief, good relief, complete relief)

For charting purposes describe patient responses in the progress notes or calculate a follow-up score by reducing the pre-intervention score by the corresponding percentage of relief.

0%	10%	25%	50%	75%	100%
No Relief	Minimal Effect	Some Effect	Good Effect	Excellent Effect	Complete Relief

WILDA credti: Fink, R.

F I G U R E   4 – 2 : Massachusetts General Hospital Pain Assessment & Reassessment (M-PAR) procedure guide.

In addition to changes in pain intensity, the nurse also should assess for any undesired effects of the treatment, such as sedation or nausea. Benefits associated with analgesia, such as enhanced activity, better participation in therapy, or improved mood or sleep also are noted. The timing of reassessments is important and ideally should be done at the anticipated time of the "peak effect" (15 to 30 minutes after IV morphine, 60 minutes after oral immediate-release morphine) whenever possible, or within the window of the "duration of action," such as within 4 hours of administration of a short-acting oral or parenteral dose of morphine.

Pain Assessment in Specific Populations

Although pain assessments are individualized, there are specific populations who are at risk for having their pain undertreated or untreated because of mistaken beliefs or unwarranted fears. It was not too long ago when nurses and other health professionals believed that children could not feel or remember pain. Older adults were believed to have dulled senses that lessened pain awareness. Neurologically or chemically impaired patients were thought to have no awareness, physiological consequences, or subsequent memory of pain. Chronic pain was believed to be a mental illness, with reports of pain being a call for attention or for some secondary gain. Patients with an addiction disorder were believed to report pain only to secure the drugs needed for their next "high." It was erroneously believed that the risks of using local anesthetics, or analgesics far outweighed any possible benefits in each of these populations. Research and clinical practice in this area informs us that pain can be experienced, assessed, prevented, and should be safely relieved in virtually all of these patient groups. Developing advanced pain assessment skills will help the nurse challenge these outdated (but prevalent) notions and prevent the useless pain these vulnerable populations often endure.

Pediatric Patients

It is now accepted that anatomic, physiologic, and biochemical elements necessary for pain transmission are present in newborns, regardless of their gestational age. The American Academy of Pediatrics and the Canadian Paediatric Society compel all professionals [15] to do everything possible to prevent, reduce, or eliminate pain in children, especially neonates. Pain is known to cause short-term physical and psychosocial harm in children; especially for neonates. Although physiologic stress is a major concern with unrelieved pain, physical measures, such as a change in vital signs, make for poor, unreliable indicators of pain. Behavioral observation and surrogate reporting by those who know the infant or child best are the recommended methods for assessing pain in the preverbal child.

Facial expressions, body movement, and cry are the most widely used measures of pain for the full-term infant [16, 17]. The classic picture (see Fig. 4–3) of the pained facial expression in infants includes the following:

- Medial, inferior movement of eyebrows creating a vertical furrow (bulge) between them
- Eyes tightly shut
- Cheeks raised creating a groove between the nose and upper lip
- Wide-opened mouth forming a square

The cry of pain has been distinguished from other cries by its sudden onset and loud, high-pitched cry without preliminary moaning, followed by periods of breath-holding [17]. Behavioral responses, such as withdrawing from pain; or physiological measures, such as a transient 20% spike in heart rate and blood pressure, have been integrated into some measure of pain during infancy [18].

Children may be less able than adults to articulate experiences or needs related to pain, which may result in undertreated pain. However, some 3-year-olds can accurately report the location and intensity of their pain. Behavioral measures, such as the FLACC Scale, which rates **f**acial expressions, **l**eg movement, **a**ctivity, **c**ry, and **c**onsolability, may be used for children up to 7 years old (see Fig. 4–4), who are unwilling or unable to reliably self-report the presence and nature of their pain [19, 20]. Behavioral measures in

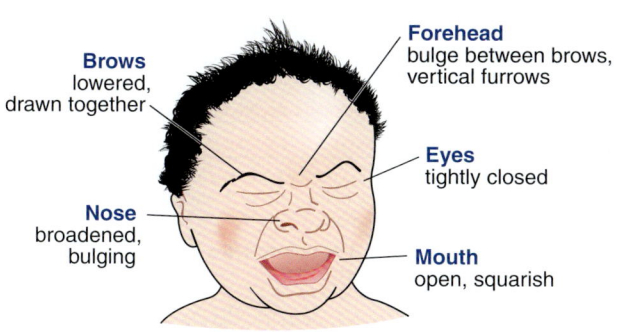

FIGURE 4–3: Face of pain in an infant.

Revised - FLACC (Face, Legs, Activity, Cry, & Consolability) Scale

Face:
0 = No Particular Expression or Smile
1 = Occasional grimace or Frown, Withdrawn, disinterested
2 = Frequent to constant frown, clenched jaw, quivering
   Individualized behavior*:_____

Face Score: _____

Legs:
0 = Normal position or relaxed
1 = Uneasy, restless, tense
2 = Kicking or legs drawn up
   Individualized behavior*:_____

Legs Score: _____

Activity:
0 = Lying quietly, normal position, moves easily
1 = Squirming, shifting back and forth, tense
2 = Arching, rigid or jerking
   Individualized behavior*:_____

Activity Score: _____

Cry:
0 = No cry, awake or asleep
1 = Moans or whimpers, occasional complaint
2 = Crying steadily, screams or sobs, frequent complaints
   Individualized behavior*:_____

Cry Score: _____

Consolability:
0 = Content, relaxed
1 = Reassured by occasional touching, hugging or talking to, distractible
2 = Difficult to console or comfort
   Individualized behavior*:_____

Consolability Score: _____

Total Score: _____

*Individualized expressions of pain may be noted in each category and ranked according to frequency or intensity of the behavior, particularly for those with cognitive impairment.

0 = Comfortable; 1–3 = Mild discomfort; 4–6 = Moderate pain; 7–10 = Severe pain/discomfort

FIGURE 4–4: Revised Face, Legs, Activity, Cry, & Consolability (FLACC) Scale.

children will not detect pain in the child with atypical presentations (e.g., stoic or withdrawn behaviors) or the child who lays motionless, appearing to sleep in response to pain [21]. Children more than 4 years of age can use crayons or colored markers to locate pain on a body diagram, or can use other tools, such as the Faces Pain Scale (see Fig. 4–5) or OUCHER scales developed for this population. Multidimensional pain scales have been developed for the assessment of children with recurrent or chronic pain and generally are used by pediatric pain specialists [21].

Older Adult Patients

Although it is a myth that pain is an inevitable part of aging, persistent pain is more common among older adults than cohorts of other ages. Studies have shown that about one-half of those older than age 65 experience pain that has lasted for at least a year [22], and more than two-thirds of institutionalized elders have pain that is often untreated.

Pain in older adults interferes with ambulation and socialization and has been linked to depression and high utilization of costly health-care services [23]. Despite this, it may be difficult to evaluate pain in the older adult because of physical and mental changes associated with aging, or values and beliefs about pain. Pain may be intense if nerves have been sensitized from previous unresolved pain; whereas other times, significant tissue damage (e.g., silent heart attack) may occur without pain being

These faces show how much something can hurt. This face (point to left-most face) shows no pain. The faces show more and more pain (point to each from left to right) up to this one (point to right-most face) – it shows very much pain. Point to the face that show how much you hurt (right now).

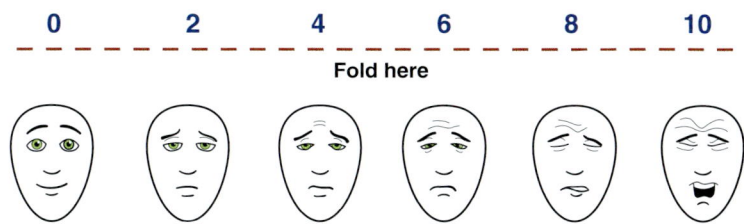

FIGURE 4–5: Revised faces pain scale. Numbers are not made visible when the scale is presented to patients. Versions in other languages available from: http://www.painsourcebook.ca.

experienced. In some situations, pain presents itself with atypical symptoms, such as confusion, restlessness, or irritability. This is especially true in patients with dementia, who have a difficult time understanding and verbalizing what they are feeling [24].

As for patients in other age groups, self-report of pain is the gold standard for assessment. The Numeric Rating Scale, Verbal Descriptor Scale, and Faces Pain Scale are the most established tools for the alert, cognitively intact older adult; although simply worded questions are the most effective. The revised Faces Pain Scale is the tool for measuring intensity preferred by older adults, including those who are from ethnic minorities or those with mild-moderate cognitive impairment [24]. For patients with considerable cognitive impairment or those with dementia, tools have been validated to quantify their pain using behaviors, such as facial grimace, vocalizations (e.g., moaning), body movements (e.g., rubbing), interpersonal changes (e.g., irritability, aggressiveness), and changes in usual activities (e.g., sleep or eating patterns).

Although there are a few behavioral pain assessment tools developed for this population, there is a lack of consensus about the best one to measure pain in all patients. Pain Assessment in Advanced Dementia (PAINAD) tool rates pain on a 0-to-10 scale based on breathing, vocalizations, facial expressions, body movements, and consolability [25] (see Fig. 4–6). However, this instrument will miss or underestimate pain in patients whose presentation of pain is manifested as a change in daily activities, interpersonal interactions, or mental changes. Therefore, adding surrogate reporting of pain by people who know the patient best or observing the response to empirical treatment with analgesics has merit in this population [26].

PAINAD (Pain Assessment IN Advanced Dementia)

	SCORE
Breathing: 0 = Normal 1 = Occasional labored breathing. Short period of hyperventilation. 2 = Noisy, labored breathing, periods of hyperventilation; Cheyne-Stokes.	
Negative Vocalizations: 0 = None 1 = Occasional moan/groan. Low level, disapproving quality speech. 2 = Repeated troubled calling out. Moaning, groaning, crying.	
Facial Expression: 0 = Smiling or inexpressive. 1 = Sad, frightened, frown. 2 = Facial grimace.	
Body Language: 0 = Relaxed. 1 = Tense, distressed, pacing, fidgeting. 2 = Rigid, fists clenched, knees pulled up. Striking out. Pulling or pushing away.	
Consolability: 0 = No need to console. 1 = Reassured or distracted by voice or touch. 2 = Unable to console, distract, or reassure.	
TOTAL SCORE	

* One or more points suggest the presence of pain with higher scores or surrogate reporting from those who know the patient validating it. Higher scores suggest more severe forms of pain are being experienced.

F I G U R E   4 – 6 : Pain Assessment IN Advanced Dementia (PAINAD).

 NURSE-TO-NURSE TIP

Patients who are comatose, severely brain-damaged, intubated, or chemically paralyzed, cannot display signs of pain. However, after emerging from these states, patients have informed clinicians that pain can be perceived, produce suffering, and be recalled. Physiological signs often are invalid although respiratory effort (see Fig. 4–7) may signal pain [27]. Nurses must assume pain is present (APP) and treat it in these patients when they have conditions associated with pain (e.g., bone fractures, cancer, or nerve damage) or undergo procedures known to be painful (e.g., suctioning, chest-tube removal) even if unresponsive [28].

Critical Care Pain Observation Tool

Indicator	Description	Score
Facial Expression	0 = Relaxed: Neutral facial expression 1 = Tense: Frowning, brow-lowering, orbit tightening, &/or levator contraction 2 = Grimace: All of facial criteria above plus eyelids tightly closed	
Body Movements	0 = Absence of movements: (does not necessarily mean no pain) 1 = Protection/guard, withdraws: Slow, cautious movements, rubs pain site 2 = Restlessness/thrashing: Pulls tube, attempt to sit, climb out of bed, thrash, strikes out	
Muscle Tension Evaluate w/ passive flexion/ extension of arms	0 = Relaxed: No resistance to passive arm movement 1 = Tense, rigid: Resists to passive arm movement 2 = Very tense, rigid: Strong resistance to passive movement	
Ventilation Compliance or Vocalization (if extubated)	**Ventilated Patient** 0 = Tolerating ventilator, no alarms 1 = Intermittent alarms, stop spontaneously, coughing 2 = Fight ventilator/asynchrony, frequent alarms **Extubated, "vocal" Patient** 0 = Quiet/normal tone 1 = Sigh, moaning 2 = Crying out, sobbing	
	TOTAL:	

Instructions for use:

Observe the patient's face and body movement at rest and rate those aspects accordingly. Observe for vocalizations (if extubated) or compliance with ventilator and score per the appropriate scale. Passively move the patient's arms and rate the level of resistance to body movements on a 0-2 scale.

Add up the scores for each measure to determine a total score. Scores of >1 at rest indicate the presence of pain. Scores >2 with movement (turning) indicate pain. Higher scores generally provided more support for the presence of severe pain, but the relationship is not linear (a 4 is not twice as intense as a "2") and a low score (e.g. "2") can indicate the presence of severe pain.

FIGURE 4-7: Critical care pain observation tool.

Patients with Chronic Pain

Patients with unrelenting chronic pain may suffer intensely and report very high levels of pain intensity with few or inconsistent behavioral signs. Chronic pain affects the body, mind, spirit, and social relationships in an undesirable way, making it particularly important to have the patient distinguish the physical and psychosocial components of pain separately [1].

Physically, the pain limits functioning and contributes to the disuse and deconditioning that further interferes with activities of daily living and role functioning. The extent of functional impairment is a better measure of disease severity and the effectiveness of treatments than changes in the "pain score" alone [29]. Patients with chronic pain are asked to report the most pain, least pain, and average pain over the past month. This helps to establish variability over time and may reveal patterns useful in guiding treatment or lifestyle changes (see Fig. 4–8).

Mentally, individuals with chronic pain may change their outlook, becoming more pessimistic, often to the point of helplessness and hopelessness. Mood often becomes impaired when pain persists, as the sadness of being unable to do important or enjoyable activities, combined with self-doubts and learned helplessness escalates the risk of depression. The anxiety surrounding the timing of pain flares, as patients worry about their physical ability to do what is needed; the uncertainty about coping with multiple competing demands can escalate to the point of panic.

Spiritually, chronic pain may be perceived as a punishment for wrongdoing, as a betrayal by the higher power, as a test of fortitude, or as a threat to the essence of the patient, resulting in shattered dreams and a disrupted sense of purpose. Socially, pain often strains valued relationships due to the impaired ability to fulfill role expectations, which places burdens on others. Chronic pain affects the essence of the person, thus disturbing every aspect of his or her life. A comprehensive assessment (see Fig. 4–8) should therefore explore the physical, mental, spiritual, and social changes that have occurred since the onset of his or her chronic pain. Probes designed to reveal pertinent thoughts, feelings, insights, activities, coping styles, and relationships help pain specialists identify therapeutic targets.

A noteworthy point is that therapeutic encounters are a form of social interaction. When caring for patients with chronic pain, the nurse becomes part of their pain experience. A self-awareness of values and nonverbal communication can facilitate the establishment of an accepting and nonjudgmental milieu. As a nurse, paying attention to subtle aspects of the relationship may restrict passivity and encourage independent (active

Comprehensive Pain History for Chronic Pain Patients

Patient ID: _____ _____   Date: _____

Character of primary discomfort
(Circle all that apply)

Sharp	Cramping	Burning
Aching	Throbbing	Stabbing
Soreness	Sickening	Shooting

Other:_____

Intensity of discomfort
Right now: (Use 0–10 scale below)

0	1 2 3	4 5 6	7 8 9	10
No pain	Mild pain	Moderate pain	Severe pain	Worst pain ever

Worst pain in the past month:

| 0 | 1 2 3 | 4 5 6 | 7 8 9 | 10 |

Least pain in the past month:

| 0 | 1 2 3 | 4 5 6 | 7 8 9 | 10 |

Location of Pain
Site of primary discomfort:_____
Radiation of pain:_____
Other painful areas: _____

Timing of Pain
(onset, constant/intermittent)_____
_____

Modifying Factors
Worsens pain: _____
Reduces pain: _____

Treatments
Tried, no benefit: _____
Partial, temporary relief: _____
Prolonged benefit: _____
Want to try; think will help: _____

Past/Present History of Abuse
(Circle types)

| Physical abuse | Sexual abuse | Drug abuse |

Effect of Pain on Close Relationships:
_____
_____

Effect of Pain on Activities
(Use 0–10 scale below)

0	1 2 3	4 5 6	7 8 9	10
No effect	Slight effect	Moderate effect	Major effect	Unable to do

Personal care/hygiene:

| 0 | 1 2 3 | 4 5 6 | 7 8 9 | 10 |

Work-related activities:

| 0 | 1 2 3 | 4 5 6 | 7 8 9 | 10 |

Social and intimate activities:

| 0 | 1 2 3 | 4 5 6 | 7 8 9 | 10 |

Home/family responsibilities:

| 0 | 1 2 3 | 4 5 6 | 7 8 9 | 10 |

Recreational activities:

| 0 | 1 2 3 | 4 5 6 | 7 8 9 | 10 |

Effect on Thinking
(Circle if noted)

Confusion	Forgetful	Ruminating
Self-doubts	Helpless	Acceptance
Catastrophizing	Confident	

Other (specify): _____ _____

Effect on Emotions
(Circle if noted)

Worried	Frustrated	Anxious
Scared	Angry	Depressed
Stressed	Irritable	Cared for

Other (specify): _____

Primary Sources of Stress:
_____
_____

Sources of (emotional) Support:
Who do you turn to for help? _____
What do they do that helps the most? ___
Is religion/spirituality helpful? _____

Effect of Pain on Close Relationships:
_____
_____
_____

FIGURE 4–8: Comprehensive pain history for chronic pain patients.

coping) behaviors. Overly solicitous responses or overtly punishing social interactions have been found to increase pain intensity, whereas caring or distracting exchanges have a more desirable effect on pain.

Patients with a Suspected Addictions Disorder

One serious concern shared by many nurses is the possibility they may be duped by patients who are feigning pain to get drugs to support a habit, criminal activity, or an addiction disorder. Nurses and other health professionals tend to overestimate the likelihood of drug seeking when patients are actually demonstrating relief-seeking behaviors. Often these conclusions are based on assumptions or biases rather than established assessment methods [30].

The first point of confusion is when expected pharmacological effects are misinterpreted as an addiction. The emergence of withdrawal symptoms (dependence) or the tendency to need higher doses over time (tolerance) occur with many types of medicines and should not be considered as evidence of addiction. See the definitions in Box 4–1.

Pseudoaddiction has been used to describe an understandable response to severe unrelieved pain that mimics drug-seeking or addictive behaviors [31]. Patients with pseudoaddiction, desperate for relief, are distraught while demanding that pain relievers be provided. When pain relief is not provided, the patient may escalate his or her demand for analgesics and other pain behaviors. A crisis of mistrust develops between the patient and caregivers that undermines the therapeutic process. Not knowing where else to turn, formal complaints may be filed while maladaptive behaviors escalate to aggressive, illicit, or deceptive actions [32]. The distinguishing feature of pseudoaddiction is that these behaviors go away when the pain is relieved.

The hallmark signs of an addiction disorder are excessive craving, compulsive use, and continued use despite known harm [30]. An addiction disorder is a treatable brain illness that precludes the ability to exercise proper judgment or experience normal pleasures. Along with displacing

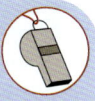

COACH CONSULT

Social responses to patients in pain have been categorized as solicitous, punishing, or distracting in nature. Solicitous responses of providing more assistance than is necessary can actually increase the patient's pain and reduce independent functioning. Punishing responses (e.g., getting mad when pain is reported), increases emotional distress and may push patients to act in a way that risks injury. Distracting and caring responses acknowledge the pain and then help shift attention toward coping or healing activities.

Box 4–1 Definitions Related to Addictive Disease*

- **Physical dependence:** Adaptation that is manifested by a drug-class–specific withdrawal syndrome, which can be produced by abrupt cessation, rapid dose reduction, decreasing blood level of the drug, and/or administration of an antagonist.
- **Tolerance:** A state of adaptation in which exposure to a drug induces changes that result in a diminution of one or more of the drug's effects over time.
- **Pseudoaddiction:** An iatrogenic syndrome created by the undertreatment of pain. It is characterized by patient behaviors, such as anger and escalating demands for more or different medications, and results in suspicion and avoidance by staff. Pseudoaddiction can be distinguished from true addiction in that the behaviors resolve when pain is effectively treated.
- **Addiction:** A primary, chronic, neurobiological disease with genetic, psychosocial, and environmental factors influencing its development and manifestations. It is characterized by behaviors that include one or more of the following: impaired control over drug use, compulsive use, continued use despite harm, and craving.

*Adapted with permission from a consensus document developed by the American Pain Society, American Academy of Pain Medicine, and the American Society of Addiction Medicine [33a].

 NURSE-TO-NURSE TIP

Recognizing signs of opioid withdrawal are important to prevent discomforts and complications. They include:
- Yawning, insomnia
- Sweating, chills, rhinorrhea
- Anxiety, restlessness, tachycardia
- Dilated pupils, piloerection
- Nausea, vomiting, diarrhea
- Abdominal pains, other pains

These can first be noted as early as 6 hours after the last dose of a short-acting opioid, such as morphine or oxycodone or as long as 96 hours following the last dose of methadone. Remember, withdrawal is evidence of physical dependence, not addiction.

natural "reinforcers," such as food, family, and friends, drugs of abuse also eventually lose their ability to gratify, placing the addict on a compulsive quest for more drugs and for greater drug potency as their reward circuitry becomes increasingly blunted and desensitized.

Too often nurses fail to confront the patient and conduct a focused assessment or document behaviors suggestive of addiction. They may jump to inaccurate conclusions about whether or not the patient has an addiction disorder. There are several interview questionnaires and physical examination approaches to identifying aberrant drug behaviors and addiction disorders with which nurses should be familiar. In most cases, patients will be forthcoming if questions are asked in a direct and respectful manner. In contrast, they may become uncooperative and deceptive if disrespected [33] or labeled. Avoiding the question is counterproductive, as patients often do not volunteer information, especially if their disclosure may be used to limit access to necessary care.

A nurse can use simple, direct questions about illicit drug use and about past or current use of alcohol or drugs on a regular basis. Questions, such as, "Do you drink alcohol?" and "What drugs have you taken in the past month?" are good preliminary questions. Follow-up questions to affirmative responses should delineate the specific quantity and pattern of consumption using a calm, nonjudgmental, respectful approach. The CAGE-AID is a simple set of screening questions that have been expanded to identify abusers of alcohol or drugs [34]. The Opioid Risk Tool is a five-item interview guide based on known risk factors predictive of problematic drug-related behaviors.

There are a variety of validated questionnaires successfully being used to screen patients before prescribing opioids for pain [35, 36]. However, the reality remains that no set of questions is perfect nor guarantees complete honesty. Innovations in abuse-deterrent formulas and prescription monitoring programs make it more difficult for the abuse or criminal diversion of opioids, but again, no system developed to date is perfect. Applying a one-dimensional solution (focusing on the drug) is unlikely to fix a multidimensional problem. Multiple strategies (i.e., screening, monitoring, drug selection, counseling) are becoming a standard part of the way patients requiring opioid therapy are assessed and treated (see Table 4–3).

In addition to questioning patients, the nurse should purposely look for signs or behaviors suggestive of a drug abuse problem, specifically:

- Signs of intoxication
- Lesions (track marks) and swelling along veins

COACH CONSULT

Assessing and relieving pain in patients with addictive disease challenges nurses to set aside related prejudices and develop advanced skills. Unrelieved pain increases stress and drug craving. Inadequate pain management may contribute to relapse in the recovering patient or increased drug use in the patient who is actively using. Nurses have a duty to relieve pain and provide humane care to all patients, including those patients known or suspected to have addictive disease.

Table 4–3	**Behaviors That are More or Less Predictive of an Addiction Disorder**	
MORE PREDICTIVE OF ADDICTION	**LESS PREDICTIVE OF ADDICTION**	
Selling or stealing prescription drugs	Reporting psychic effects (getting high)	
Crushing, injecting, or snorting oral drugs	Unsanctioned dose escalation	
Losing prescriptions repeatedly	Aggressive complaining	
Current abuse of illicit drugs	Request specific drugs	

- Erosions of the nasal septum
- Changes in personality, social habits, or role functioning

These signs are likely to be known by persons closest to the patient. Signs associated with opioid effects (i.e., sedation, constricted pupils, and slurring of speech) or withdrawal (i.e., yawning, sweating, dilated pupils, tachycardia, and abdominal pains) may not signal a problem for a patient who has been prescribed opioids but would be concerning in a patient who denies taking opioids. Denial is a common sign of addiction, a clearly intoxicated patient (with no evidence of a neurological disorder) who denies drinking or drugging raises a red flag. Urine drug screens provide an additional source of information capable of revealing aberrant drug behaviors. Drug screens, however, can be imprecise and fail to identify opioid diverters (those who sell drugs) and addicts; or they can wrongly label persons as such. For example, a person who inadvertently eats poppy seeds may test positive for morphine [37]. When used properly, drug screens can improve the ability to guide treatment and advocate for patients.

When cutting through the facts, myths, uncertainties, and attitudes surrounding concerns about pain and addiction, there are a few principles that nurses should remember:

- The majority of pain patients do not have an addiction disorder, nor an intent to sell drugs
- Drug abuse is prevalent in our society
- Prescription pain relievers are among the most commonly sought and abused substances

- Nurses have a duty to meet the health and comfort needs of individual patients
- Nurses have a duty to protect society by limiting access to controlled substances [38, 39]

Screening for substance abuse disorders is a small but important part of a systematic pain assessment (see Box 4–2). Nurses developing the assessment skills required to identify aberrant drug behaviors fulfill a necessary component of a balanced approach. In addition to preventing opioids from being diverted to the illicit market, pain must be treated when it is present, even in a patient with an addiction disorder.

Box 4–2 Principles of a Systematic Pain Assessment

- Pain must be assessed in all patients and reassessed after interventions
- Pain is always subjective; patient report is the gold standard for measurement
- Nurses have a duty to accept self-reports unless clear reasons for disbelief exist
- Pain has both physical and emotional components that can be evaluated separately
- Physiological/behavioral signs of pain; or surrogate (nurse or family) pain ratings are unreliable and should be used only when the patient is unable to self-report
- The WILDA method reminds nurse to ask about words, intensity, location, duration and aggravating/alleviating aspects of pain
- Other symptoms and the effect of pain also should be evaluated
- Pain can exist without a definable source, however a physical assessment should search for a treatable cause
- Special considerations are needed when assessing pain in different populations who have difficulty or are unable to self-report pain
- Nurses should assume pain is present in paralyzed or unconscious patients who have conditions or procedures known to be painful
- Jumping to conclusions about problems and motivations of patient with chronic pain or substance abuse disorders should never replace focused assessment

5 Diagnoses, Treatment Planning, and Refinement

DX and TX

CHAPTER 5

Diagnoses, Treatment Planning, and Refinement

The General Process of Relieving Pain

Caring for a patient with severe unrelieved pain can be a daunting task for nurses. The process can be simplified by following steps of the nursing process and critically analyzed by asking related questions (see Box 5–1). First, the nurse assesses the patient to identify physical problems generating pain and psychosocial and spiritual factors influencing its perceived intensity. Next the nursing diagnosis and realistic comfort/function goals are delineated within the context of the patient's overall health and expected trajectory. Pharmacological and nonpharmacological agents are tailored based on the pain intensity and type and patient preferences. Given unpredictable individual responses, even the best-planned treatment strategies need to be evaluated for immediate and delayed-onset effects, and then modified.

In addition to standard nursing processes, pain care is optimal when:

- The therapeutic environment is patient-focused
- The professional teams' and patient's goals are mutually developed and in alignment
- Multimodal techniques, including different medication and nondrug therapies are used
- Attentive monitoring and treatment refinements are tailored based on individual response

Given that successful treatment of pain can determine whether the nurse-patient relationship is frustrating or mutually rewarding; attentive care planning is an endeavor worthy of effort. This chapter will review the steps of the nursing process with emphasis on developing and tailoring the treatment plan to best meet the individual's needs.

Box 5–1 Checklist of Critical-Thinking Questions Using the Nursing Process

Assessment
- Has a comprehensive assessment been completed and documented? Is the type of pain (acute, chronic, neuropathic, etc.) clear?
- Are findings by different professionals consistent?
- Who else might provide reliable information?
- What does the patient want and need?
- Are there needs or values in conflict with others involved in the care?

Diagnosis
- What are the actual and potential nursing diagnoses?
- What nursing diagnoses are the highest in priority?
- What diagnoses are related to each other?
- Are the relational statements and manifestations clearly stated?

Outcome Identification and Planning
- What are the patient's goals for comfort and function?
- Are the expected outcomes for this patient realistic?
- Are therapeutic goals of doctors, nurses, and the patient aligned?
- What interventions are to be used?
- Who is the best-qualified person to perform these interventions?
- How involved can the patient be at this time?

Implementation
- What pharmacological agents are available?
- Is there flexibility in the timing and dose of analgesics?
- What doses and dosing intervals have been used?
- Have enough doses been administered (consistently) to reach steady state?
- What treatment-specific safety precautions are needed? What culturally-based factors need consideration?
- What nondrug pain relief methods has the patient used in the past?
- What nondrug pain relief measures is the patient willing to learn or try?
- What pain amplifiers (e.g., inflammation, distress) can be targeted?

Evaluation
- Were the interventions successful in achieving comfort/function goals?
- Is therapy safe and efficacious?
- Has therapy been tailored to the individual's needs, preferences, and responses?
- What parts of the treatment plan are modifiable?
- Are there barriers undermining the effectiveness of care?
- What can be done to promote communication, collaboration, and continuity of care?

Assessment of Pain

Assessment of pain is the foundation upon which the treatment plan is built. Lacking knowledge of the presence or nature of pain; will likely lead to analgesic gaps and treatment failures. Inherent in effective pain treatment planning is a need to tailor the approach based on individuals' needs and responses. It may be useful for the nurse to think about acute pain as a "drive," such as hunger or thirst. Once the underlying need is met, the discomfort subsides and is no longer the focus of attention. As such, pain is signaling an underlying necessity, which the analytical nurse uncovers and addresses as part of therapy. There may be a series of basic needs contributing to the pain, such as the requirement to:

- Identify and treat the underlying illness/injury causing the pain
- Change a pattern of behavior causing repetitive stress or strain
- Identify and manage emotions that can amplify pain
- Resolve inner (spiritual, developmental) or outer (role expectation, cultural) conflicts
- Adjust lifestyle patterns, such as nutrition, exercise, sleep, and/or stress levels

In contrast, chronic pain may be related to errant signals in the pain-processing centers. As such, there may be no cause-directed cure, and no underlying requirement to be satisfied. The psychosocial factors listed above are relevant and important aspects of pain, regardless of the type. Refer to Chapters 2, 3, and 4 for details pertaining to:

- Conducting a comprehensive pain assessment
- Distinguishing acute from chronic pain
- Distinguishing somatic, visceral, and neuropathic sources of pain
- Identifying triggers, amplifiers, and dampeners of pain

In addition to assessing a patient's current pain, evaluating his or her previous pain experiences is equally important.

The patient's beliefs about what will relieve the pain strongly influences expectations and actual responses to the interventions provided.

Nursing Diagnosis

After assessment, the next step in the nursing process is establishing a nursing diagnosis. The nursing diagnosis helps identify and prioritize actual or potential health problems that demand nursing attention. The process of diagnostic reasoning entails:

- Developing the diagnosis based on assessment
- Validating the diagnosis with the patient, family, and other health-care providers
- Prioritizing the individual patient's need(s)
- Documenting in a way that helps determine realistic outcomes and a plan of action

The process of establishing a nursing diagnosis of pain is straightforward when patients can verbalize their discomforts and related information. Definitions established by the North American Nursing Diagnosis Association (NANDA) [1], include:

- Acute Pain: Severe discomfort with a duration of less than 6 months
- Chronic Pain: Severe discomfort with a duration of more than 6 months

The diagnostic statement typically specifies location, and etiological factors, when known. Nurses improve the usefulness of their diagnosis by adding diagnostic clues to the statement. For example, a nursing diagnosis statement "Acute postoperative pain," can be expanded to: "Acute incisional pain; manifested by facial grimace and refusing to move or deep breathe."

Because the presence of pain can affect so many aspects of a person's life, pain may be the source of other nursing diagnoses. Examples of such nursing diagnoses follow:

- Ineffective Airway Clearance related to incisional pain manifested by weak cough
- Hopelessness related to feelings their chronic pain will never end
- Anxiety related to anticipated pain similar to a past experience with poor pain control
- Ineffective Coping related to chronic back pain, avoidance of activity or problem-solving
- Knowledge Deficient of effective (drug and nondrug) pain-relief interventions
- Impaired Physical Mobility related to arthritic pain in knee and ankle joints
- Disturbed Sleep Pattern related to increased pain perception at night

Goal Setting

The process of goal setting and outcomes identification is a more involved and integrated process than establishing the diagnosis. Whenever possible, this step secures input and agreement among patient, family, and health-care providers. Additionally, the process involves:

- Establishing objective, measurable, culturally appropriate outcomes
- Predicting expected benefits, weighed against foreseeable costs and risks
- Aligning goals with
  - Patient values
  - Realistic expectations
  - Available resources
  - Environmental, situational, and ethical constraints
- Estimating a time line for attainment of expected outcomes
- Documenting the goals and updating them based on response

The Nursing Outcomes Classification (NOC) system provides a structure to guide the establishment of goals based on objective, measurable criteria [2]. This system delineates desired outcomes from the *nursing perspective* as:

- Minimal adverse psychological responses
- Consistent pain control
- Minimal life disruption secondary to pain
- Pain level controlled to the extent that behaviors and vital signs are uncompromised

These outcomes focus on preventing the mental confusion, fear, anger, helplessness, and despair that accompanies uncontrolled pain. Desired outcomes also focus on minimizing the interference of pain with usual daily routines, responsibilities, and important relationships.

Desirable patient-centered outcomes are best delineated when they represent objective, measurable goals the patient says he or she would do if pain was satisfactorily controlled, such as:

- Get out of bed and walk for 5 minutes, 2 times tomorrow
- Be comfortable and steady enough to stand and shower
- Fully participate in today's physical therapy for 30 minutes
- Play a family game of Scrabble without yelling or falling asleep

Inherent in many of these goals is the need to find a balance to ensure that neither the pain, nor the side effects of medications are interfering with physical, mental, or social functioning.

Establishing Realistic Expectations

Pain reduction remains an important goal, without setting the expectation that pain will be eliminated. If patients hurt while expecting "no pain," it is natural to feel scared and angry. The person may fear something is wrong, perhaps a missed diagnosis or a botched procedure. Anger naturally results when there is a mismatch between expectation and reality, or when the patient feels he or she was treated unfairly. Therefore, when setting comfort/function goals and patients express "no pain" as their expectation, nurses need to educate and counsel them on the following:

- A pain-free state, while desirable, may not be achievable
- The reduction of pain intensity by 30% to 50% is more achievable than eliminating it
- There is a need to balance concerns between pain reduction and functional improvement
- Responses to pain medicines vary and it takes time to find the best combinations/doses of medications with the fewest possible side effects

These messages convey a clear expectation with a subtle undertone that the nurse's responsibility is not to "take away the pain." Instead, nurses work with patients, who actively participate in their care (to the extent possible) to promote comfort, functioning, and the achievement of additional treatment goals. Nurses also communicate with family members and the treatment team, so that collective goals and expectations can be aligned.

Treatment Planning

Basic treatment strategies vary based on pain type, duration, and expected trajectory. **Acute pain** is prevented or aggressively treated to promote recovery and prevent nerve sensitization that intensifies and prolongs pain. **Chronic pain** therapy includes treatments that target the underlying chronic disease to the extent possible. If interventional, surgical, and/or medication management strategies yield only partial or temporary relief; the focus of treatment shifts to promote the highest possible level of functioning, coping, and quality of life despite the persistence of pain. At the **end of life**, planning focuses on the quality of time spent with family and friends while ensuring that the dying process is as comfortable and dignified as possible. Also at the end of life, pain may be just one of a cluster of uncomfortable symptoms. When dealing with symptom clusters, treatments are planned to select medicines that lower pain without worsening other bothersome symptoms. Regardless of the pain type, planning uses the principles of multimodal therapy to address the pain and the underlying problem or process, including biopsychosocial and spiritual needs.

Planning to Meet Physical Comfort Needs

Plans to meet the physical needs of patients with pain include drug, nondrug, and environmental interventions to promote comfort and healing. Patient's comorbid conditions and medications are taken into account to prevent adverse events related to drug-drug or drug-disease interactions. The history of a patient's prior exposure to pain and analgesic medications is an important consideration when planning to meet his or her needs. These personal experiences may have:

- Altered his or her sensitivity to pain
- Created anxiety or fear surrounding the experience of pain
- Revealed how particular analgesics work for him or her
- Taught him or her helpful nondrug pain-relief techniques

For mild, intermittent pain, this can be accomplished with nondrug measures and nonopioid analgesics on an as-needed basis. For moderate or severe pain, multimodal pharmacological therapy is the cornerstone of treatment. Whenever pain is severe enough to require opioids, NSAIDs and/or adjuvants can be added for their synergistic and opioid-sparing capacity. Additionally, when opioids are indicated, the distinction between an opioid naïve and an opioid-tolerant patient is important to consider when establishing a safe, effective therapeutic plan. For neuropathic pain, adjuvant medications may be the mainstay of treatment with analgesics added on an as-needed basis.

A variety of nondrug pain relief approaches should be integrated into the plan. These can further lower analgesic requirements or be used at times of analgesic gaps. This helps reduce pain, anxiety or fear, and helplessness triggered by not knowing what to do when pain flares. When analgesic gaps are unavoidable, nondrug methods can be combined to target different pain components simultaneously, for example:

- Icing and compressing cutaneous targets that **transduce** pain
- Suppressing spinal pain **transmission** through postural alignment and positioning
- Relieve distressing emotions capable of amplifying (**modulating**) pain
- Distract attention away from the **perception** of pain with music or humor
- Patient education and counseling regarding helpful interpretations and **responses** to pain

Since the time of Florence Nightingale, nurses have appreciated the important influence that environment has on patient responses. It is well known that bright lights and loud noises worsen headaches, and perhaps other pains [3, 4]. An unfamiliar environment, such as a hospital, with its noises, bright florescent lighting, unpleasant odors, and hurried activity, can compound pain. Nurses can alter environmental stimulation in a way that lessens its negative affect on pain.

Planning to Meet Psychosocial Comfort Needs

Cognitive, emotional, and social factors influence the perception and ability to control pain. Knowing what the patient believes will work for his or her pain is important as that information influences a person's expectations and actual response to the interventions provided. Helping patients know what to expect goes a long way toward alleviating fear and anxiety that can drive pain levels up. If a patient has unrealistic negative expectations, it is important to challenge and correct this type of thinking, which can contribute to anxiety, fear, helplessness, and depression.

During the planning stages, nurses educate patients about how pain is assessed and anticipated treatments to relieve it. Education about patient-controlled analgesia or implanted devices is most effective while the patient is alert, and before he or she actually needs to use judgment to operate it properly. This education often is integrated into preadmission educational materials.

Patient and family education about the pain treatment plan is important when they are responsible for adhering to it in the community. Caregiver beliefs also can affect their willingness to support the regimen and assist the patient. Patients and caregivers need to understand:

- Underlying causes of pain, its anticipated trajectory, and the intent/duration of therapy

- Proper storage and handling of drugs and devices
- How and when to implement treatments
- Treatment's desired effect
- Warning signs that must be reported to health-care providers
- Lifestyle changes demanded by the treatment (e.g., eating pattern, restricted alcohol, driving)
- Effect treatment may have on daily activities (e.g., bathing) or role (e.g., working)
- Who to call if the drugs are ineffective or cause side effects
- Dangers of unauthorized dose adjustment or sudden cessation of therapy

It is well known that anxiety, fear, and other distressing emotions are capable of driving pain levels up. Providing more opioid or NSAID medication does nothing to quiet these pain amplifiers. Specific methods of reducing emotional arousal and alleviating these emotions will help decrease their pain and suffering.

Patients in pain respond differently to the social environment based on the nature of their pain and personal preferences. Some people prefer to withdraw when they are in pain, whereas others prefer the distraction of people and activity around them. Nurses may need to limit the type, number, and length of time that visitors may stay with the patient, respecting his or her preference. Alternatively, they may coordinate resources and adjust the environment to provide needed stimulation and distraction. The quality of social interaction also matters to those with pain. For instance, toddlers tolerate pain more readily when supportive parents, child life specialists or nurses comfort and distract them. Conversely, a child may lie motionlessly in pain, pretending to sleep [5], when strangers are nearby.

Socially, pain often strains valued relationships, in part because of the impaired ability to fulfill role expectations. In turn, this can produce stress, conflict, and perhaps a family crisis. Pain may be endured as a sacrifice for loved ones, such as the single parent who ignores substantial pain to stay on the job to support his

COACH CONSULT

Pain strains family relationships. Caregivers who feel frustrated or burdened can be counseled and allowed to "vent" *privately* their concerns, such as how pain interferes with role functioning, family finances, companionship, and intimacy. In the patient's *presence* the nurse can demonstrate adaptive interactions that avoid solicitous or punishing responses while distracting attention from pain. Nurses can mobilize family strengths to facilitate communication, expressions of love, problem-solving, and to gain commitment needed for treatment plan adherence.

or her children. Numerous factors can affect a person's perception of and reaction to pain. The nurse who takes time to know these aspects of the individual is in a better position to tailor an effective treatment plan, making a lasting contribution to the person's comfort, health, and well-being.

Planning to Meet Spiritual Needs

To the extent that pain affects the essence of the person, it can be a source of spiritual distress and suffering, or be a source of strength and motivation. As such, this distress can amplify or diminish the intensity of pain. Planning to meet patient's spiritual needs can be challenging until the nurse knows the patient's innermost concerns, values, and the endorsed meaning of his or her life. This sense of spirituality may or may not be religious in nature; although as part of planning, the patient is asked if he or she has spiritual needs or religious preferences that should be honored.

Interventions

After the plan of care is developed, nurses are responsible for its implementation to the best of their abilities. See Chapters 6, 7, and 8 on pharmacologic management, nondrug, and invasive treatments for details. Despite the requirement for medical orders, nursing judgment often is needed to select from different analgesic options, and determine doses needed within the confines of a range order. Nurses can plan a patient's care in a way that provides an analgesic around the clock (ATC), and supplements with prn doses for spikes in pain and during painful (e.g., dressing changes, physical therapy) procedures. If analgesia is ordered on a prn basis, nurses can offer analgesics as soon as they are due for patients who have pain that is expected to last for hours or days. This relieves pain before it becomes severe, and while it is more responsive to analgesia. This effort to "stay ahead of the pain" prevents neurological changes that spread, intensify, and prolong pain; while facilitating the attainment of a pharmacological steady state. Research [6] supports that administering analgesics ATC rather than prn results in fewer side effects, better relief, and greater patient [6] satisfaction, because patients feel:

- Less like a complainer or a burden to nurses
- More in control, able to refuse medication if they do not need it
- Less worried about whether or not the medicine is due
- Less worried about drug abuse or becoming "a junkie" [6; p. 641]

Nondrug pain relief methods also should be offered routinely. These can include a variety techniques described in Chapter 7, or what the patient has found useful in the past. Patients often respond with less pain, lowered emotional distress, and better coping when these methods are tried. Instead of replacing medications, these techniques complement analgesics, helping fill analgesic gaps while waiting for a dose to work, or to help cope with breakthrough pain not adequately relieved by medication.

If a patient has an analgesic infusion device or other pain-relieving technology, it is the nurse's responsibility to ensure the equipment is properly set up and functioning as intended. On transfer between units and at change of shift, nurses verify the infusion pump settings against the order. Nurses also routinely evaluate the insertion site and system integrity in a systematic fashion from patient to the medication source. They also check for the integrity of alarms (e.g., not silenced) and the connection to a power source.

ALERT !

A careful history of exposure and responses to analgesics in the past reveals vulnerabilities to adverse medication effects. Stomach aches from nonprescription analgesics elevate the risk of NSAID-induced gastrointestinal (GI) ulcerations or bleeding. Those with asthma and nasal polyps may develop anaphylactic reaction to aspirin-like products. Opioid-naïve patients who became sleepy after weak opioids need vigilant monitoring for respiratory depression when given opioids. Comorbidities, such as hypertension, renal insufficiency, lung disease, obesity, and sleep apnea also elevate analgesia-specific risks.

Refinement to the Plan Based on Reassessment

Even the best planned and executed interventions may not satisfactorily alleviate pain and suffering. Vigilant monitoring and reassessment of the patient during and after pain-relief interventions is vital because of unpredictable responses. Evaluation of the interventions need to be systematic, ongoing, and criterion based [7]. The assessment section (Chapter 4) delineates 3 essential conponents of reassessment as:

- Analgesia—how much the pain was reduced
- Activity—how much activity and ability to participate in therapy was affected
- Adverse events—the development of undesired effects or complications of therapy

The nurse should consider what is working, what is not working, and what has yet to be tried. Some organizations have flow diagrams (see Fig. 5–1) to provide decisional support about the methods and resources

Pain Assessment/Management Decision

Screen for Pain on Admission

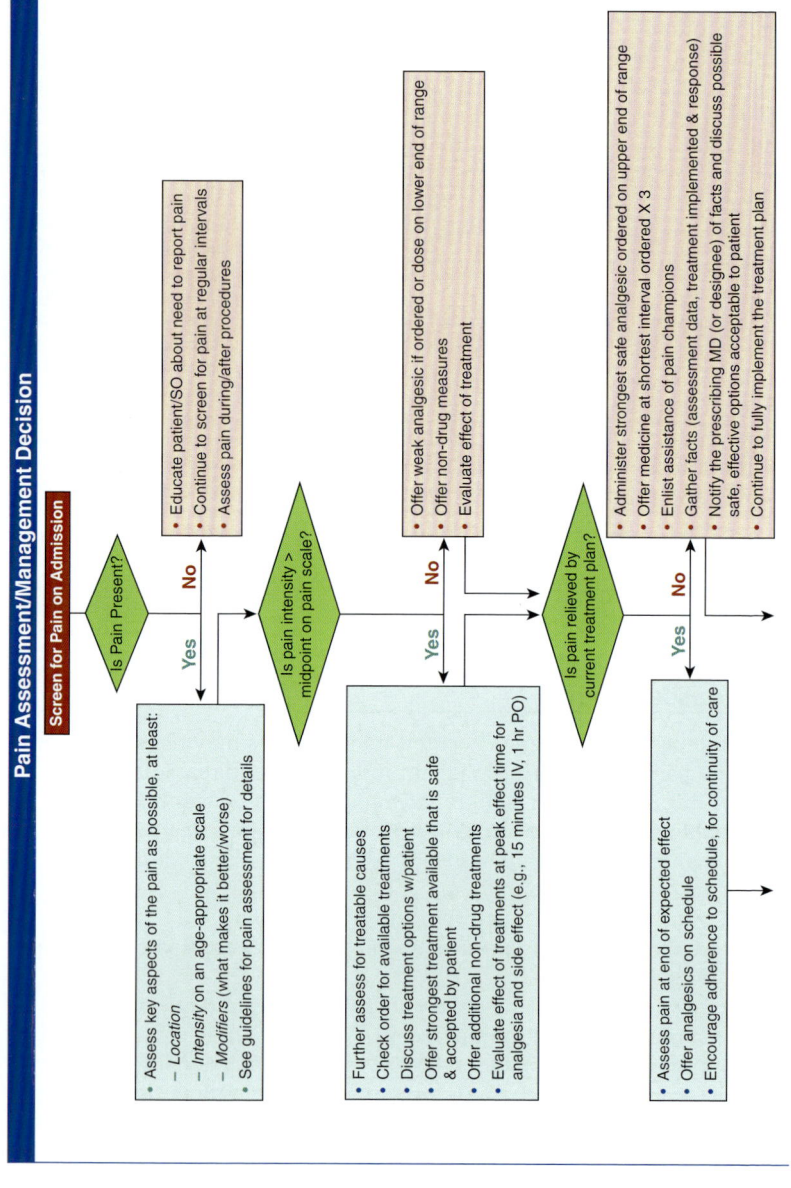

Is Pain Present?

No →
- Educate patient/SO about need to report pain
- Continue to screen for pain at regular intervals
- Assess pain during/after procedures

Yes →
- Assess key aspects of the pain as possible, at least:
  - *Location*
  - *Intensity* on an age-appropriate scale
  - *Modifiers* (what makes it better/worse)
- See guidelines for pain assessment for details

Is pain intensity > midpoint on pain scale?

No →
- Offer weak analgesic if ordered or dose on lower end of range
- Offer non-drug measures
- Evaluate effect of treatment

Yes →
- Further assess for treatable causes
- Check order for available treatments
- Discuss treatment options w/patient
- Offer strongest treatment available that is safe & accepted by patient
- Offer additional non-drug treatments
- Evaluate effect of treatments at peak effect time for analgesia and side effect (e.g., 15 minutes IV, 1 hr PO)

Is pain relieved by current treatment plan?

No →
- Administer strongest safe analgesic ordered on upper end of range
- Offer medicine at shortest interval ordered X 3
- Enlist assistance of pain champions
- Gather facts (assessment data, treatment implemented & response)
- Notify the prescribing MD (or designee) of facts and discuss possible safe, effective options acceptable to patient
- Continue to fully implement the treatment plan

Yes →
- Assess pain at end of expected effect
- Offer analgesics on schedule
- Encourage adherence to schedule, for continuity of care

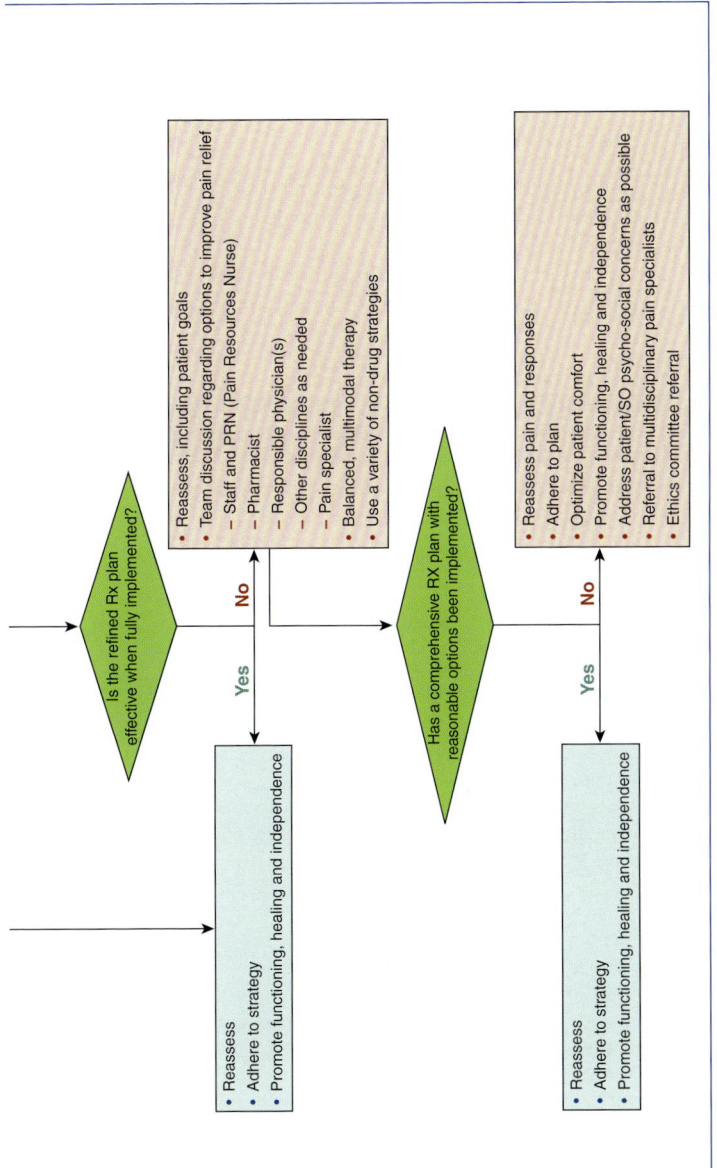

FIGURE 5–1: Sample pain-treatment planning, decision tree.

available to facilitate the treatment planning process. Other questions to consider in a systematic stepped approach to reassessment and refinement of therapy are delineated in Box 5–2. The following questions also should be considered:

- What is the underlying need?
- What type of pain needs treatment?
- What type of distress needs to be reduced?
- What are realistic comfort/function goals?
- What are the analgesic options?
- What are potential nondrug pain-relief options?
- What adjustments may be needed based on response?

Box 5–2 Steps and Questions for Reassessment and Treatment Plan Refinement

Step 1: Review assessments, treatments provided, and responses.
- Have new or different diagnoses emerged?
- Is the patient's goal for comfort and functioning realistic?
- What barriers to pain relief have been identified? Which have been addressed?
- What emotional distresses have been identified? Which have been addressed?

Step 2: Analyze the alignment of the treatment with the pain type.
- Are non-opioids being used for mild pain, aching, or as part of multimodal therapy?
- Are mixed/weak opioids being used for moderate pain?
- Are strong opioids being used for severe pain?
- Are adjuvants directed at the cause; or for calming pain-generating nerves?
- Have medications been administered consistently enough to achieve a steady state?

Step 3: Consider the merit of changing the regimen, discuss with pharmacist and prescriber.
- If ineffective or not tolerated, has switching the drug been considered?
- Has a dosage adjustment been tried?
- If effective intermittently have adjustments been tried?
  - Scheduling around the clock rather than prn dosing?
  - Long-acting agent tried for constant pain with a known effective dose?

Step 4: Implement the refined analgesic regimen.
- Are analgesics consistently offered on schedule?
- Are there 2 or more consecutive ratings below the pain scale midpoint?

- Does dose adjustment +/– 25%–50% achieve acceptable levels of comfort/side effects?
  - Work within limits of range order or secure revised order.
- Add coanalgesics/adjuvants as ordered to target multiple mechanisms and cut side effects.
- Document interventions and timely evaluations of responses to guide further refinement.

Step 5: Use nondrug techniques to complement the analgesic regimen.
  - Have a variety of techniques been tried?
  - Has the technique the patient believes to be most effective been tried?
  - Does reducing emotional distress also reduce pain levels?

Step 6: Access available resources (e.g., pain specialists) and referrals for advanced techniques.

Whereas a comprehensive pain assessment is an integral part of planning treatments, the interpretation of how pain changes over time and responds to therapy is an essential part of refining the treatment plan. In hospitals, consistent documentation of the nature and intensity of pain on a well-crafted flow sheet can promote continuity of care and fine-tuning of the treatment plan. In outpatient or community-based settings, having patients keep a pain diary is useful, especially when pain is chronic. A pain diary is typically completed 3 times daily, at set times, allowing for pattern identification and treatment evaluation. The format of diaries may vary, but basically include:

- Date, time, and setting
- Intensity and description of physical sensations and emotional distress
- Factors that worsen or improve pain
- Actions taken to relieve discomforts

Professionals periodically review the diary entries with the patient to gain insight into factors that can cause, exacerbate, or alleviate pain [8–10]. Specific factors that are analyzed include:

- Consistent time of day or night when pain is best or worse
  - If always worse at night, a change in evening medication or activity may help

- Specific day of the week that is best or worst
  - If always best on weekend, weekday patterns are explored and modified
  - If weather makes a difference, create a plan for coping with those exacerbations
- Concordance between high/low levels of the sensation and distress parts of pain
  - Be sure patient has treatments and coping skills for both sensations and distress

Patterns that lead to improvement in pain may not be apparent immediately, but consistent use and guided interpretations help patients develop understanding and skills in refining treatments.

It also is important to identify any potential barriers to pain treatment that might undermine therapy. The patient's reluctance to report pain or concerns about developing an addiction are the most common problems encountered. Nurses should directly address these barriers by informing patients and significant others:

- Pain is an important part of treatment to discuss with nurses when experienced
- Pain can be treated without causing addiction
- Any concerns about addiction should be discussed openly and honestly with professionals

Adjustments to Pharmacological Treatments

Given unpredictable individual responses to standard doses of specific medications, most patients will require an adjustment to the dose or interval between doses. Often a change of the dose or interval by 25% to 50% up or down is sufficient for the desirable response. Whereas nonopioid drugs have a ceiling dose above which no additional analgesic effects are realized, opioid drugs can continue to be titrated upward cautiously, while monitoring for respiratory depression or other unacceptable side effects. If the selected analgesic fails to provide relief at the maximum tolerated doses, then switching to another agent is warranted. Switching to another medication in the same class often promotes tolerability and efficacy, with strategies for doing this safely described in the pharmacology section (Chapter 6).

Many common side effects of analgesics can be managed with pharmacological or nondrug methods (see Table 5–1). With NSAIDs, gastroprotection is most important, especially with high-dose therapy, or when used for more than several days. With ongoing NSAID therapy, periodic

Table 5–1 Treatment of Common Analgesic Side Effects

SIDE EFFECT	DRUG THERAPY	NONDRUG THERAPY	COMMENT
NSAID-Induced Gastritis or Peptic Ulcer	Proton-pump inhibitor (lansoprazole) Prostaglandin E replacement (misoprostol) with precautions for childbearing women	Take with food, milk, or antacid first. Drink 8 oz. water after. Avoid alcohol. Avoid other GI irritants.	Use enteric-coated formulations when available. Note weight gain or swelling with history of heart failure.
Constipation	Stimulant laxative (senna or bisacodyl), alone or with stool softener (docusate) Osmotic laxatives (lactulose, polyethylene glycol, sorbitol) Saline laxative (magnesium citrate or milk of magnesia) Methylnaltrexone bromide Enemas	Increase fluid intake (e.g., 36–48 fluid ounces water/day). Increasing fiber and exercise may help.	Constipation persists demanding a bowel regimen for duration of opioid therapy. Laxatives usually needed. Fentanyl patch is less constipating than oral oxycodone or morphine.
Nausea and Vomiting (N/V)	Antihistamines (meclizine, diphenhydramine) especially if worse when walking. Antipsychotics (haloperidol, prochlorperazine) Prokinetic agents (metoclopramide) Serotonin antagonists (ganisetron, ondansetron)	Eliminate unpleasant sights and odors. Small, frequent meals. Cool, bland foods (limit spices, fat, fiber) Restrict liquids. Loosen clothes, recline after eating with fresh air or fan	Tolerance to emetic effect develops after several days of opioid therapy. Try reducing antiemetics over time. May need to change the drug or dose of analgesic used.

Continued

Table 5–1 **Treatment of Common Analgesic Side Effects—cont'd**

SIDE EFFECT	DRUG THERAPY	NONDRUG THERAPY	COMMENT
Pruritus	Antihistamine (e.g., cetirizine, diphenhydramine, loratadine) Nalbuphine, a mixed agonist-antagonist opioid may help. Serotonin 5-HT(3) receptor antagonists, NSAIDs, and dopamine (2) receptor antagonists being studied.	Apply cool packs, lotion, and diversional activity.	Most likely a side effect, not allergy. Tolerance to itching develops over several days. More common with spinal opioids.
Urinary Retention	Antihistamines may help. Usually adjust dose, change agent, or route. Discontinue other anticholinergic drugs.	Encourage to void every few hours. May need to catheterize.	More common in men with spinal routes of analgesia.
Sedation	Caffeine, dextroamphetamine Methylphenidate, Modafinil Reduce dose and shorten interval or change route.	Stimulation of senses.	Observe respirations. Tolerance develops. Restrict dangerous activities and driving.
Respiratory Depression	Opioid antagonist, naloxone hydrochloride (Narcan) Oxygen	Stimulate, prompt breathing. Stop opioid. Life support prn.	If coadministered with a sedative, flumazenil may be given.

screening for GI bleeding, elevated liver enzymes, impaired renal functioning, and hypertension should be performed. With opioids, transient problems of nausea and vomiting can be controlled with short-term antiemetic therapy. Constipation however, continues for the duration of opioid therapy, requiring ongoing prophylaxis and treatment. With sustained opioid therapy, periodic screening is done for long-term endocrine, neurological, or behavioral effects.

Coanalgesic medications, such as antidepressants or antiepileptic drugs may produce sedation, dizziness, or other side effects. These drugs are typically initiated at subtherapeutic doses and are titrated slowly over a matter of weeks as the patient develops tolerance to the undesired effects. Some of the older coanalgesics (e.g., amitriptyline and carbamazepine) may carry a higher side effect burden and require monitoring for toxicity compared with newer agents. Topical agents, such as the lidocaine patch 5%, can develop local skin irritation but are generally free from systemic side effects or toxicity. Increasingly, drug manufacturers are developing pain relievers that have better safety and efficacy, use less invasive routes of administration, and pinpoint novel targets. Additionally, more sophisticated monitoring equipment is being developed to detect these side effects before they pose a threat.

Other refinements to the pharmacological treatment plan may be made based on the individual's circumstance. For example if a dressing change involving a vacuum-powered dressing is painful, the suction can be shut off an hour before the dressing change to allow some moisture to accumulate, facilitating its removal. Additionally, a topical or analgesic systemic can be administered so that its peak action coincides with the scheduled dressing change. If pain consistently awakens the patient, interrupting sleep, a long-acting opioid or a continuous opioid infusion at night may help. When patients use PCA devices, they may need to be prompted a few times during an hour, to reinforce teaching about how repeated small doses may be used to reach the desired level of analgesia. Subsequently, less frequent doses are needed to remain comfortable.

Adjustments may be made to the nondrug therapies as well. Adjustments may be based on the patient's willingness to try new methods, or mastery of techniques learned. In contrast, adjustments may be needed because new problems emerge as a result of maladaptive responses to pain. For example, excessive immobility, disuse, and deconditioning often are driven by fear avoidance, learned helplessness, and/or low self-efficacy beliefs. The patient becomes too scared to move, that produces weak, stiff, tense muscles that spasm with activity; which positively reinforces the fear-avoidance cycle. Nursing interventions that calm, educate, encourage, guide, and direct patients to do specific activities can improve their activity levels. Nondrug interventions such as heat, massage, pacing of activities, and enhancing self-efficacy will help lower pain, while improving mood and function.

Finally, refinements are made to the treatment plan over time as the patient recovers and his or her pain-relief needs change. Often hospitalized postoperative patients follow a predictable course. Following a period of high-potency parenteral or spinal analgesics, there is a transition to oral opioids on the second or third postoperative day when pain subsides. Additionally, doses are reduced over time, dosing intervals become longer and eventually most patients can change to intermittent dosing with opioids when something stronger than nonopioids is needed. Over a period of a few weeks, most patients will require only intermittent NSAID therapy.

Case-Based Examples of Treatment Planning and Refinement

Sample case-based discussions are presented here as examples of the critical-thinking process behind pain treatment planning. This is not intended to be comprehensive, rather, just touch upon some types of pain and populations that require special considerations.

Acute Pediatric Bone Fracture

Consider the case of Jimmy Nee, a 3-year-old who broke his right tibia jumping on a trampoline. Pain was evident and Jimmy could tell the nurse while pointing to the right knee "it hurts a lot." Behavioral indicators (FLACC scale) score his pain 9/10 when moving and 5/10 when at rest. He has no other medical conditions and takes no medication. His parents are with him, and able to console him. When the doctor told him she will need to straighten his leg just a little and put a cast on, Jimmy screams and yells, "don't touch my leg, it will hurt." The doctor decides to start an IV to administer medications and provide fluids. The parents inform the nurse that Jimmy hates needles. Planning for Jimmy's pain treatment needs, the nurse considers the following:

- What is Jimmy's underlying need?
  - Fractured leg bone needs brief manipulation and casting
  - Activity restriction during and after the procedure
- What type of pain needs treatment?
  - Pain related to needlestick and reduction/casting procedure
  - Acute somatic pain secondary to fracture and muscle spasm
- What type of distress needs to be reduced?
  - Anxiety regarding the procedural pain and the casting procedure
  - Fear of needles
  - Fear of pain when injured leg is touched

- What are realistic comfort/function goals?
  - Control pain and fear enough to be casted without further injury
  - Analgesia for a few days to support nighttime sleep and daytime (restricted) activity
- What are the analgesic options?
  - Topical numbing medicine before needlestick for IV insertion
  - Systemic opioid and anxiolytic for the closed reduction/casting procedure
  - Postprocedural nonopioid
- What are potential nondrug pain relief options?
  - Icing before and after procedure
  - Breathing techniques, guided by blowing bubbles
  - Distraction techniques (TV, DVD movie, pop-up books)
  - Child life specialist input into language to use when describing procedure to Jimmy
  - Play therapy with a casted teddy bear
- What adjustments may be needed based on response?
  - Ensure venipuncture site is numb before insertion is attempted
  - Balancing safety and efficacy of procedural sedation and analgesia

Discussion of Plans for Controlling Jimmy Nee's Pain

Preliminary pain treatment is planned based on knowledge of Jimmy's age, gender, presence and involvement of parents, and reported prior responses ("hates needles") to pain. Parental involvement will be sought to help lower anxiety and coach Jimmy in the use of non-drug relief measures. As with all children, age-appropriate medicines with weight-based dosing will be used to determine the specific opioid and dose needed before and during the reduction/casting procedure and for the nonopioid recommended after the procedure. Close monitoring for safety and efficacy will be in place whenever a sedative and opioid are used concurrently. Aspirin is avoided in children, and some orthopedic specialists prefer acetaminophen over NSAIDs following a bone fracture to minimize bleeding and suppression of the inflammatory phase of bone healing.

Jimmy will need interventions to prevent pain anticipated for two types of painful procedures. Environmental, nonpharmacologic, and pharmacologic interventions can be used to prevent, reduce, or eliminate pain [11], anxiety and fear; resulting in short-term and long-term benefits [12]. For the venipuncture, topical local anesthetics are indicated, whereas for a fracture reduction and casting procedure systemic opioid analgesia with

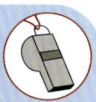
anxiolysis or sedation will be required. The topical local anesthetic product selection may be dictated by the timing of the procedure. EMLA (lidocaine 2.5%/prilocaine 2.5%) cream can take up to an hour to work and cause venous constriction making inserting the venous catheter more difficult. L.M.X.4 (lidocaine 4%) cream works in 30 minutes, whereas rapid onset topical anesthetics, such as ethyl chloride spray, or J-tip devices can be used moments before a painful procedure. Nondrug methods may be used concurrently but during the actual procedure, distraction, breathing, and affirmations are best.

Young Athletic Woman with Acute Postoperative Pain

Maria Los Turnia, a 20-year-old redheaded woman who fell while she was competing in a national championship downhill skiing event, injuring her knee. The MRI confirmed a sprained left knee and she is admitted to the Orthopedic Day Surgery Center for reconstruction of the torn ligament. Her health has been otherwise excellent with no medications, although she drinks nutritional supplements and takes many vitamins. She is distraught over losing this tournament, but determined to return to compete for a spot in the next Olympics. Postoperatively, she must be admitted to the hospital because of severe, uncontrollable pain. The aching and throbbing in her knee is rated at 10/10, is unresponsive to 20 mg IV morphine given over 2 hours, and prevents her from using the continuous passive motion device or getting out of bed.

- What is the underlying need?
  - Remove pain as an impediment to her recovery
  - Monitor for complications (bleeding, compartment syndrome) that present as severe pain
- What type of pain needs treatment?
  - Acute postoperative pain on top of acute traumatic pain
- What type of distress needs to be reduced?
  - Grieving loss of tournament, anxiety regarding future competitions

- What are realistic comfort/function goals?
  - Cut pain by 50% to allow participation in rehabilitation
  - Prevent pain sensitization and musculoskeletal deconditioning
- What are the analgesic options?
  - Multimodal therapy including high-dose opioids, NSAIDs, and adjuvant medication
  - Continuous epidural infusion or femoral nerve block
- What are potential nondrug pain-relief options?
  - Icing through a Cryo-Cuff device, positioning for comfort
  - Relaxation, imagery, affirmations, distraction
  - Reduction of sources of distress/suffering
- What adjustments may be needed based on response?
  - Rapid titration, adjustment in medications to terminate pain crisis

Discussion of Maria Los Turnia's Pain Treatment Plan

Effective perioperative pain management strives to prevent pain before it occurs or can escalate to severe intensity. This "preemptive analgesia" involves the administration of local anesthetic, systemic opioids plus an NSAID and/or an adjuvant pain reliever (e.g., gabapentin) just before, during, and after surgery. Additional nondrug measures, such as icing the surgical site, music, affirmations; or administering energy-based healing techniques (e.g., Reiki) add value to the pharmacological approaches [13]. It is unclear from the case description which of these were done preoperatively, however this combination should be implemented as soon as possible to prevent the windup and sensitization of nerves that occurs with severe pain.

As a redheaded woman, her metabolism may be such that she needs more or a different type of anesthesia and analgesia than people of other genetic makeups [14–18]. Given the lack of response to high doses of morphine for an opioid-naïve patient, she should be switched to another opioid, such as hydromorphone or fentanyl, in combination with other medication and nondrug methods mentioned above. Dosing should be consistently provided either continuously or with scheduled doses for the 5 half-lives needed to reach steady state.

COACH CONSULT

Treating the recovering athlete armed with a "no pain no gain" philosophy. Recovering athletes often demand quick restoration of functioning. Aggressive use of physical modalities (i.e., ice, exercise, and electrical stimulation) to speed recovery should be tempered by the need to prevent further injury with long-term functional consequences [23].

Research [17–22] delineates gender differences in pain and response to analgesics. Women are more sensitive to pain, and have more painful conditions than men. Women are almost twice as likely to experience side effects of analgesics (e.g., respiratory depression, nausea, and vomiting) than their male counterparts. Hormonal levels, body fat distribution, and electrolyte balances may explain some differences, but not why traditional analgesics favor men while partial kappa agonists (i.e., nalbuphine, butorphanol, and pentazocine) favor women. Emerging research is detailing genetic markers accounting for the wide variation in responses to particular medications and range of doses required to alleviate pain. Initial medication selection, dose, and dose-interval adjustments may someday be based on gender, hair color, race, metabolic enzymes, and other genetic factors.

Non-English–Speaking Man with Chronic Pancreatitis Suspected of Drug-Seeking Behavior

Imin Mustafa is a 30-year-old male with a limited command of the English language. He is admitted for a flare-up of his chronic pancreatitis after his sixth emergency department visit in a week. He presents each time asking for a shot of Demerol. When transport arrives to transfer him to an inpatient room, he refuses admission claiming he will lose his job with one more absence. He wants a shot so he can make it to work in 2 hours. The doctor cancels the admission orders instead asking for 300 mg intramuscular (IM) Demerol be administered that may be repeated once in 1 hour.

The dosage is questioned and confirmed by the doctor who cites Imin's large (> 300 pound) body size, and tolerance from using 300 mg (75 mg QID) oral meperidine daily for 3 months as justifying that dose. If he is not well enough for discharge after two injections, he will be admitted for further tests and treatment. He is alert with no difficulty breathing, with equal, brisk reflexes bilaterally in all extremities. He points to his left upper-abdominal quadrant and reaches around to his mid-upper back to indicate the location of his pain. A nurse colleague asks you to give the shot to "this drug seeker."

- What is the underlying need?
  - Analysis of chronic pancreatitis to identify underlying cause (e.g., gallstones)
  - Distinguish if behavior represents aberrant drug seeking or relief seeking

- What type of pain needs treatment?
  - Visceral pain, chronic pain
- What type of distress needs to be reduced?
  - Fear of loss of work
- What are realistic comfort/function goals?
  - Relieve pain and disease exacerbation so he can return to work
- What are the analgesic options?
  - Parenteral opioids
  - Surgical or block procedures may be considered
- What are potential nondrug pain relief options?
  - Relaxation, imagery, distraction, prayer
  - Dietary restriction until symptoms improve
- What adjustments may be needed based on response?
  - Switch to another drug

Discussion of Mr. Mustafa's Plan for Immediate Relief of Chronic Pancreatic Pain

The dose of 300 mg of parenteral meperidine is likely inappropriate and unsafe. Although the rationale presented was that he is tolerant to the effects of 300 mg meperidine, his oral dose of 75 mg taken at one time is equivalent to less than 20 mg of parenteral Demerol. The explanation that his excess weight justifies the 300 mg dose also can be refuted. Whereas weight-based dosing is common for children and adults less than 50 kilograms, dose adjustments for obese patients rarely exceed 20% more than the standard starting dose. The 300 mg dose is 400% higher than the standard 75-mg starting dose. Obesity is a risk factor for serious opioid-induced respiratory depression, further suggesting the ordered 300-mg dose is unsafe. When administered via the IM route, there is unpredictable absorption and the effects of the first 300 mg may not be known within an hour when the high dosage can be repeated. Additionally, when 600 mg of meperidine is given in a day, there is a high risk of seizures, especially in a person who has been taking meperidine for more than 48 hours. Mr. Mustafa's brisk reflexes may be an early indication of normeperidine-induced neurotoxicty that causes seizures. Combined, these concerns must be presented to the prescriber to develop a safer treatment plan.

Given his status as a foreign-born person with a limited English vocabulary, secure the services of a certified health-care interpreter who speaks Arabic and can inform the team of strategies aligned with culturally sensitive care. Having an interpreter would allow the team to ask specific questions needed to verify the medical diagnosis and determine whether or not a substance abuse disorder exists. Although Imin is asking for medication

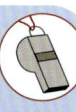
to relieve his pain, this alone is insufficient evidence of a drug problem. While awaiting the arrival of the interpreter an oral or IV opioid (not meperidine) can be administered. This will help the pain and will not worsen a substance abuse disorder if one is present.

IM injections should be avoided because they hurt, damage tissue, and produce unreliable absorption and distribution of pain medications. Meperidine combined with either Phenergan (promethazine) or Vistaril (hydrodxyzine) is known to produce tissue and fat necrosis that can be a source of long-term pain.

Chronic Arthritis Pain in an Older Adult

Arthur Rytus is an 84-year-old man with long-standing osteoarthritis of the right thumb and both knees. He presents with fatigue, shortness of breath, and a change in his stools. He is subsequently diagnosed with anemia and a gastric ulcer from NSAID use. His complete metabolic panel blood test fails to identify other problems. He is scheduled for a return visit to test for *H. pylori* as a possible cause for his ulcer in a week. His medications include amlodipine for high blood pressure, atorvastatin for elevated cholesterol, cardioprotective aspirin and over-the-counter (OTC) naproxen (Aleve) for his joint pain. He reportedly hates taking medicine, and keeps meticulous records of all his pills. During discharge teaching he is very upset that the doctor has stopped everything except the amlodipine, and strictly prohibits the use of aspirin or OTC pain relievers. Prescriptions are added for a once daily omeprazole to treat his ulcer and once daily tramadol (Ryzolt) for pain. Arthur is worried that he will get "hooked" on the pain medicine. He confides in the nurse that life is not worth living since his pain has limited his ability to visit friends at the community center and even to fill out crossword puzzles at home.

- What is the underlying need?
  - Pain reliever with a lower side effect burden than NSAIDs
- What type of pain needs treatment?
  - Chronic somatic pain

- What type of distress needs to be reduced?
  - Upset over change in medication
  - Fear of addiction to pain relievers
  - Sadness over loss of functioning
- What are realistic comfort/function goals?
  - Pain reduction to increase mobility enough for a weekly community center visit
  - Be able to complete crossword puzzles
- What are the analgesic options?
  - Weak systemic opioid
  - Topical pain relievers
- What are potential nondrug pain-relief options?
  - Herbal or nutritional supplements
  - Distraction
  - Topical warmth or aqua therapy
- What adjustments may be needed based on response?
  - Medication or dose adjustment to maximize relief, and minimize side effects

Discussion of Safe, Effective Analgesics for Mr. Rytus

Although upset about the medication change, Arthur states he hates taking medication and ends up taking only three medications per day instead of four. The dose of tramadol is started at about half of what a younger adult would start at with a reevaluation and scheduled titration in 1 week if needed in the absence of dose-limiting side effects. Mr. Rytus can be reassured that tramadol has a low risk of abuse and is not classified as a "narcotic" by the U.S. Drug Enforcement Administration (DEA). Older adults often are open to the use of topical creams or ointments. For this man's osteoarthritis, a local anesthetic or capcaisin product would be the best starting point. If those trials fail, topical diclofenac may be an option after the gastric ulcer heals. Older adults also respond well to a variety of nondrug techniques, including distraction by music, pictures, or stories that promote reminiscence of happy times during their lives. Adaptative equipment will help Arthur pursue his hobbies, including Internet-based crossword puzzles, which do not require him to write in small boxes. The Arthritis Foundation has many resourses and helpful guides for Arthur.

To help Arthur overcome his sadness related to a sense of helplessness, activities and interactions designed to enhance his self-efficacy will be beneficial. Nurses can be mindful to take every oportunity to promote independence, and challenge his pessimistic comments as untrue or unhelpful. Self-efficacy can be enhanced through nursing interventions [25–28] including:

- Verbally persuading a patient to do a specific activity
- Sharing experiences of others, in similar situations, who succeed with specific strategies
- Providing feedback related to physiologic states
- Lowering arousal levels (e.g., anxiety, stress)
- Developing skill mastery

Coordination of Care and Collaboration

Nurses hold an important collaborative role in the coordination and implementation of pain treatment plans. The optimal practice model for this activity is the interdisciplinary team model that values the expertise and insights of all professionals. Patient and family's needs remain the focus within this practice model as a blending of perspectives from different disciplines reveal greater insights of those necessities. The most effective teams have ongoing dialogs that incorporate shared goals, care planning, role blending, and shared leadership, including:

- Working for common goals
- Pooling of expertise and insights
- Having a forum for direct communication and problem-solving
- Having opportunities for personal growth and development
- Being able to share burdens and offer personal support

Effective collaboration and coordination of care allows the nurse to focus on the important work of implementing a thoughtful, refined, individualized plan of care, while evaluating its effectiveness to achieve optimal patient outcomes. Despite some inherent complexities, the nursing process, principles of patient-centered care, and multimodal therapy are combined to attain pain reduction, functional improvement, and better overall health.

6 Pharmacological Management

Pharmacological Management

Introduction

Pharmacological management is the foundation of pain treatment in most settings. Science continues to search for the "perfect drug" that is safe, effective, inexpensive, and simply named; while acknowledging that no such therapeutic agent currently exists. Two classes of analgesics (nonopioids and opioids) are now available by prescription, and all carry a U.S. Food and Drug Administration (FDA) black-box warning of potential harm [1]. Even the safest pain relievers, available without a prescription, contain a warning label. All opioids are categorized by the Institute for Safe Medication Practices (ISMP) as "high alert," and their use requires risk-reduction strategies to prevent errors [2]. Patients and other professionals depend on the nurse's knowledge and skills to administer these medications in a safe, effective manner.

General Approaches to Analgesic Use

Strategies for treating pain vary depending on the type of pain, a host of patient-specific criteria, and individual response to treatment. For treatment of cancer pain, the World Health Organization (WHO) model is widely accepted. For acute pain, aggressive, short-term analgesic use prevents pain from escalating or persisting. For persistent pain, especially neuropathic pain, many adjuvant medications can be used. Adjuvant medications are used to:

- Relieve pain
- Reduce side effects

To the degree possible, treatment is directed at resolving the cause of the pain and aid healing.

The World Health Organization Three-Step Approach

The current approach to analgesia is built on a three-step approach (see Fig. 6–1) established in the 1980s by the WHO [3], which evolved into an approach known as multimodal therapy for the treatment of acute pain and cancer pain [4]. This approach has been used for chronic noncancer pain as well, but without the same degree of consensus in the medical community. In 2006, the WHO reevaluated this approach and determined that it remains sound, defensible, and relevant [5]. The principles of the WHO stepped approach are as follows:

- By the step (WHO ladder)
- By the clock
- Adequate trial of each drug

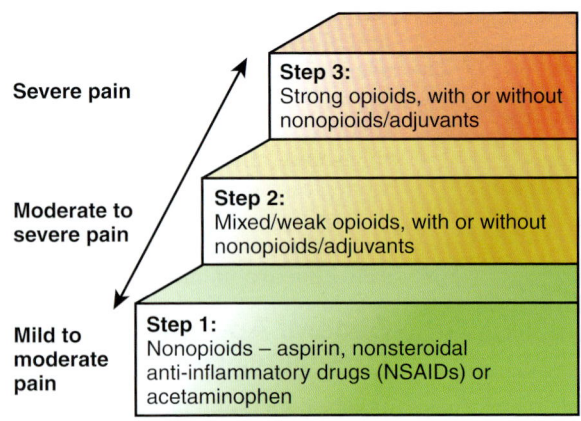

STEPPED APPROACH TO PAIN RELIEF

Severe pain

Step 3:
Strong opioids, with or without nonopioids/adjuvants

Moderate to severe pain

Step 2:
Mixed/weak opioids, with or without nonopioids/adjuvants

Mild to moderate pain

Step 1:
Nonopioids – aspirin, nonsteroidal anti-inflammatory drugs (NSAIDs) or acetaminophen

FIGURE 6–1: World Health Organization Analgesic Ladder.

- The oral route of administration is preferred, "If the gut works... use it"
- For the individual
- Attention to detail

By the Step

For patients with mild pain (1 to 3 on a 0-to-10 scale), Step 1 of the analgesic ladder, a nonopioid analgesic (e.g., aspirin) is the appropriate starting point. The nonopioid can be used with or without an adjuvant, such as a proton pump inhibitor (PPI) to reduce side effects or caffeine to enhance its analgesic benefit. If the pain persists or increases (≥4 on a 0-to-10 scale), despite the use of full doses of nonopioid medications, then a Step-2, weak-opioid analgesic such as hydrocodone is appropriate. Many Step-2 drugs, including all hydrocodone preparations contain a nonopioid (i.e., acetaminophen or ibuprofen) coingredient. If desired, a different nonopioid or an adjuvant medication can be added to the second-step regimen. If the pain persists or increases to severe (≥7 on a 0-to-10 scale) levels, then a Step-3 strong-opioid drug such as morphine, is administered and titrated. Unless contraindicated, a nonopioid and/or adjuvant medication is added to the Step-3 regimen for their opioid-sparing, pain-relieving properties. The strong opioids should then be titrated until at least a 50% reduction in pain is achieved or dose-limiting sedation and respiratory depression occurs.

COACH CONSULT

The analgesic ladder describes an upward sequence, implicitly assuming progression of disease and of pain. However, patients also may move down the analgesic ladder (e.g., after surgery). A stepped approach to coming down the ladder is indicated. For example, a progression from morphine to hydrocodone to ibuprofen is safer and more effective than switching directly from morphine to ibuprofen.

By the Clock/Adequate Trial

"By the clock" refers to the principle that analgesics need to be administered on a schedule based on knowledge of each drug's pharmacokinetic properties. For pain that is expected to continue, doses should be given at scheduled intervals around the clock (ATC), based on the duration of analgesic action. Ensuring an adequate trial of each drug, the third basic WHO principle, in part relates to pharmacokinetic properties. Medications must be given ATC for 5 half-lives of the drug to achieve a steady state in the body. Morphine, which has a half-life of 4 hr, would reach a steady state after about a day (20 hr) of ATC doses. In contrast, methadone, which has a half-life of 33 hr (±24 hr given large intraindividual variability), would not reach a steady state for a week (range of 2 to 12 days). Drugs that cause late pharmacological effects, such as reversal of inflammation or changes in synaptic receptors/chemistry, should be administered ATC for at least 1 week for an analgesic trial to be considered adequate.

Route/Individual/Attention to Detail

The oral route of administration is generally preferred because pills are inexpensive, stable, have a long shelf-life, are easy to ship and store, and are acceptable to most patients. However, some individual patients will not accept or tolerate the oral route.

For all analgesics there is great individual variability in the desired and undesired effects. The next principle, "for the individual," takes into account a variety of factors contributing to therapeutic decision making:

- Personal preferences (NOTE: patients are not "drug seekers" for stating a preference)
- Past exposure and responses to analgesics
- Demographic factors (i.e., age, gender, occupation, socioeconomic, and safety factors)
- Pharmacological needs (i.e., route, mechanism, and duration of action)
- Physiological state (e.g., comorbidities, vulnerable organ systems, ability to swallow)
- Changing individual needs and response (desired and adverse effects)

Treatment of Acute Pain

Given the time-limited nature of acute pain, there is less risk of the problems associated with long-term analgesic use, such as gastrointestinal

 NURSE-TO-NURSE TIP

Because of sporadic dosing, nurses sometimes seek to revise analgesic orders before the current regimen can be adequately evaluated. When pain persists despite prn dosing, the nurse should offer the analgesic on schedule (withholding the medication if the patient refuses or has dose-limiting side effects) or 5 consecutive doses. This will achieve a pharmacological steady state. In one study, only 5% of patients had severe pain controlled with standard prn dosing, whereas 92% had pain resolved within 24 hr when prn doses were offered on schedule. When doses are given on schedule, patients use the same amount of drugs with no more side effects, but have significantly better pain control and satisfaction during the course of their recovery [6].

(GI) bleeding or cardiovascular, renal, or hepatic effects. Acute mild or intermittent nociceptive pain (such as pain caused by bruises, strains, or superficial burn) can be treated with nonopioid analgesics on a prn basis. More severe acute nociceptive pain, such as postoperative pain or the pain caused by major trauma, typically requires at least a few days of ATC-opioid therapy. To prevent sensitization, windup, and other nervous system changes that intensify and prolong pain; an aggressive, proactive treatment approach to acute pain is advised. Acute pain arising from disorders of the viscera (e.g., angina pectoris, renal colic) requires treatment of cause, plus the selection of analgesics that are appropriate for the pain's intensity but whose side effects will not obscure the diagnosis or worsen the condition.

The **preemptive approach** treats anticipated pain. This approach involves the scheduled administration of different drugs (e.g., local anesthetics, NSAIDs, opioids, and/or antiepileptics) before and immediately after the procedure. Patients treated in this way experience less physiological stress, postoperative pain, fewer complications, and shorter hospital stays than patients who simply have anesthesia and prn analgesics after surgery. Research suggests that multimodal approaches before, during, and right after surgery yield better clinical outcomes than delayed or inadequate pain treatment [14, 15]. Successful treatment of acute pain prevents the sensitization of nerves, windup, and neuroplastic changes that amplify pain and contribute to the development of chronic pain syndromes [16].

Treatment of Chronic Pain

Once chronic pain becomes established, analgesics typically lose some of their effectiveness, even at high doses. Prolonged high-dose therapy raises

EVIDENCE FOR PRACTICE

Analgesics were once contraindicated for acute abdominal pain because it was believed that their use could lead to misdiagnosis or delayed treatment. Research repeatedly refutes this in adults and children [7–13]. Randomized, placebo-controlled trials consistently support early analgesia for acute abdomen. This approach decreases pain (50% or more) and does not interfere with diagnosis or treatment. Opioids are preferred, as they improve diagnostic accuracy, while NSAIDs may delay surgery [8, 13]. Despite this evidence, the gap between knowledge and practice remains large, and severe abdominal pain still goes untreated.

the risk of organ damage and psychosocial problems. The steps in treatment of chronic pain are as follows:

1. Treatment of the underlying disease is the first-line approach for chronic pain.
2. Analgesics with the fewest and mildest side effects. Acetaminophen often is considered first line, but may be less potent than aspirin. Topical drugs may be employed if the pain is localized and superficial in origin.
3. A multimodal approach with several medications, each with different mechanisms of action and different toxicity profiles. Adjuvant drugs may be tried at this point or during the next stage.
4. Use of opioids is best reserved for brief courses during severe flare-ups. Whenever opioids are used, a nonopioid analgesic and adjuvant drugs are used concurrently to minimize the opioid dose needed. Sustained opioid therapy may be needed in select cases.

Often several trials of different medications in each class are needed to find the medication or combination of medications that provide the optimum degree of relief with tolerable side effects. In addition to a variety of medications, different nondrug therapies, comforting techniques, and lifestyle modifications are integrated into the treatment plan.

ALERT ❗

To reduce the side-effect burden of the multimodal approach, start agents that can sedate or depress respirations at a low dose until the patient's response is observed. Patients should be warned to abstain from consuming alcohol, which can further depress respirations, and advised to not drive initially. Caution also is exercised to avoid using more than one agent (including Saint John's wort) that can elevate serotonin levels and thus pose the risk of serotonin syndrome.

Chronic neuropathic pain is particularly challenging because it results from malfunctioning or damaged nerves. Medical treatments are directed at improving the functioning of nerves, using anticonvulsants, antidepressants, local anesthetics, and/or antihypertensive drugs. Opioid analgesics may be appropriate if these drugs fail to lower the intensity of pain or improve function. Unfortunately, nonopioid analgesics are typically ineffective for neuropathic pain [17].

Pain Control at the Beginning and End of Life

Analgesic use at the beginning of life tends to err on the side of safety to avoid possible side effects. In contrast, at the end of life, side effects such as sedation may be considered a necessary part of ensuring a comfortable, dignified death. For all patients, analgesic therapy involves finding the balance between safety and efficacy.

The Perinatal Period

In the perinatal period, concerns for fetal well-being tips the balance toward the side of safety. Women may choose to use little or no analgesia during labor, with the goal of delivering a healthy, fully alert newborn. The following analgesics are considered safest in the perinatal period:

- Acetaminophen (lacks NSAID-related cardiac or bleeding effects on mother and baby)
- Mixed agonist-antagonist opioids (Nubain) may have a low risk of respiratory depression
- Carefully timed/dosed epidural analgesics (little circulating medicine reaches the fetus)

Although methadone use during pregnancy and breastfeeding is deemed safe [18], it has been studied only for women in narcotic treatment programs, not those using it for pain. The lowest effective opioid doses should be used for the shortest time possible during pregnancy, breastfeeding, and infancy. Babies born to opioid-dependant mothers are placed on a taper schedule to prevent an abstinence syndrome. The FDA warns against breastfeeding mothers using codeine as some mothers rapidly metabolize it to morphine that can result in a concentrated dose of morphine being passed on to the baby. Throughout childhood, the use of aspirin is avoided because of its link to Reye's syndrome, a fatal postinfectious encephalopathy.

The End of Life

For patients at the end of life, sedation and respiratory depression may be deemed acceptable, because the patient's comfort level is the primary concern. Pain reduction and an acceptable respiratory rate are the primary goals, while doses are sometimes increased to a level that could be considered excessive in other circumstances. Doses are administered ATC indefinitely without concern for habituation, although the nurse should control distressing side effects, such as constipation. If kidneys fail or hyperalgesia develops, patients may need to be switched from morphine or hydromorphone to a drug, such as fentanyl or methadone that does not produce potentially irritating metabolites. Sedatives may be titrated aggressively if the patient experiences agitation or refractory pain.

ALERT

On average, 27,000 acetaminophen overdoses are reported in children annually. Newborns may be particularly at risk because of the way drugs are metabolized early in life. Thus, dosing intervals are every 8 hr in neonates compared with every 6 or 4 hr respectively for infants and children (never exceed 5 doses a day). Parents need detailed instructions tailored to the product used, and the child's current weight. They should also be instructed to avoid other sources of acetaminophen.

Specific Drug Classes

Three general classes of medications are used to control pain:

- Nonopioid analgesics, including acetaminophen and NSAIDs
- Opioid analgesics, more potent than NSAIDs with morphine-like chemistry and effects
- Adjuvants, are not classified as pain relievers, but may enhance the effect of analgesics, treat discomforts other than pain, or reduce side effects. Common examples include local anesthetics, antidepressant, or anticonvulsant drugs that can prevent or reduce pain.

Nonopioid Pain Relievers

NSAIDs work by interfering with the body's inflammatory response, specifically with the cyclooxygenase (COX) cascade that occurs in response to tissue damage. Different forms of cyclooxygenase exist in the body and specific analgesics block them to varying degrees. The COX-1 form has healthy effects on platelets, the GI tract, kidneys and many other tissues. Blocking COX-1 effects is believed to cause the well-known side effects of NSAIDs (i.e., GI ulceration and bleeding, diminished renal blood flow, and inhibited clotting). Blocking COX-2 more specifically targets pain and inflammation. Drugs in this class that selectively target COX-2 chemicals are called COX-2 Selective agents, while others are sometimes referred to as "nonselective" or "traditional" NSAIDs. Table 6–1 lists the major NSAIDs and gives information on dosing, side effects, and additional nursing considerations.

EVIDENCE FOR PRACTICE

An estimated 10% to 20% of older adults are prescribed NSAIDs, which account for 3,300 deaths and 41,000 hospitalizations in the United States annually [19]. Ibuprofen has the best efficacy and GI safety among NSAIDs. Diclofenac sodium and naproxen have intermediate (doubled) risks, while piroxicam and ketorolac have the greatest (fourfold) risk of GI ulcerations or bleeds [20]. NSAIDs will worsen established hypertension or congestive heart failure.

Early research suggests cardiovascular risks in healthy patients may be greater with celecoxib and lower with naproxen. The occurrence of rare but serious cardiovascular events and skin problems prompted the FDA to request a withdrawal of rofecoxib (Vioxx) in 2004, and valdecoxib (Bextra) was later voluntarily withdrawn from the marketplace. Celecoxib (Celebrex) remains on the market, although patients with sulfur allergies should not take it, and low-dose aspirin therapy negates its gastroprotective advantage.

Table 6–1 Nonopioid Analgesics (NSAIDs)

GENERIC NAME & BRAND EXAMPLES	ANALGESIC DOSE (ADULT)	TYPICAL DOSING INTERVAL	SIDE EFFECTS AND TOXICITY PROFILE	COMMENTS
Acetaminophen (Tylenol, Datril)	325–1,000 mg (anti-inflammatory effect negligible)	q 4 hr (no more than 5 doses or 4,000 mg/day)	Minimal if any side effects. Liver and possible renal damage.	Liver toxicity limits daily dose to 4 gm per day (2 gm/day on days alcohol is consumed or with liver disease).
Acetylsalicylic acid (aspirin)	325–650 mg	qid	Among the most irritating to GI tract. Some hepatic, renal, and CNS toxicity.	Antiplatelet effect lasts 14 days. Used as cardioprotective agent. Comorbid asthma and nasal polyps may predict hypersensitivity.
Celecoxib (Celebrex)	200 mg	bid	Fewer GI side effects than most NSAIDs especially first 6 months.	Do not use w/ history of sulfur allergy, RI, HTN, or CHF.*
Choline magnesium trisalicylate (Trilisate)	750–1,500 mg	bid	Fewer side effects, less toxic than aspirin.	May be dosed 2 or 3 times a day. Less analgesic benefit than aspirin.
Diclofenac sodium (Voltaren, Arthrotec)	75 mg	bid	Some GI upset and renal toxicity.	May be dosed 2 or 3 times a day. Avoid with HTN, RI, or CHF.*

Continued

Table 6-1 Nonopioid Analgesics (NSAIDs)—cont'd

GENERIC NAME & BRAND EXAMPLES	ANALGESIC DOSE (ADULT)	TYPICAL DOSING INTERVAL	SIDE EFFECTS AND TOXICITY PROFILE	COMMENTS
Ibuprofen (Motrin, Advil)	200–400 mg (pain) 600–800 mg (pain and inflammation)	qid	Some GI upset at higher dose. Renal toxicity.	8-hr antiplatelet effect negates cardioprotective benefit of aspirin.
Indomethacin (Indocin)	25–50 mg	2–4 times daily or 1 ER/day	GI, renal, cardiovascular, skin, hematologic, and neurologic toxicity may occur.	Limit daily dose to <200 mg/day.
Ketorolac (Turadol)	20–60 mg (15 mg if >65 renal disease, or <50 kg). Maximum daily 40 mg oral or 120 mg IV	Different dosing schedules.	GI upset & bleeding, hypersensitivity, renal toxicity, and bleeding may be more severe than with other NSAIDs.	Higher loading dose then lower. Only for severe pain. Short term use (<5 days).
Nabumetone (Relafen)	1,000 mg initially, then 1,500–2,000 mg/day	Daily or bid	Fewer side effects, less toxic than aspirin	Avoid alcohol or other NSAIDs.
Naproxen (Naprosyn) Naproxen sodium (Anaprox)	220–500 mg	q12 hr	Fewer side effects, less toxic than aspirin.	May be best for cardiovascular risk. Does not negate cardioprotective benefit of aspirin.
Piroxicam (Feldene)	10–20 mg	daily	GI, renal side effects more common than other NSAIDs.	Antiplatelet effect lasts 1–3 weeks.

*GI—gastrointestinal; HTN—hypertension; CHF—congestive heart failure; RI—renal insufficiency; ER—extended release.

Individual NSAIDs have similar analgesic potency, but they vary in their anti-inflammatory properties, metabolism, excretion, and side effects (see Box 6–1 for common side-effect information). These drugs have a **ceiling effect**, meaning a dose above a certain point yields no additional relief. Therefore if a dosage is increased with no improved relief, a return to the lower dosage is recommended. NSAIDs also have a relatively narrow **therapeutic index:** a small margin between the dose that produces a desired effect and a dose that may produce a toxic effect.

Selecting, Administering, and Evaluating the Use of NSAIDs

Although notable differences exist among NSAIDs, all generally are quite effective in treating mild pain or discomforts described as "sore" or "aching." NSAIDs are avoided immediately after a bone fracture, laceration repair, or orthopedic surgery as the anti-inflammatory action can theoretically interfere with healing. Emerging research suggests bone healing is not impaired by transient use of NSAIDs in the immediate post-trauma or postoperative period, however many orthopedic surgeons continue to avoid their use.

When used in combination with opioids for moderate or severe pain, NSAIDs produce an additive effect that is considered opioid-sparing. Ibuprofen has replaced aspirin as the model drug in this class because most people tolerate it better. No NSAID has proven to be a better analgesic than ibuprofen. Ketorolac, the first parenteral NSAID, has been marketed as being comparable (in a small single-dose trial) with an opioid. When tested against ibuprofen, it failed to prove its superiority [21]. The GI toxicity of ketorolac limits therapy to no more than 5 days.

There may be specific conditions that respond better to particular NSAIDs (e.g., aspirin for sunburn, indomethacin for gout), but these drugs

---

Box 6–1 NSAID Awareness: Gastrointestinal Side Effects

The most common side effect of NSAID is GI irritation, such as heartburn and indigestion. These occur because NSAIDs inhibit the production of prostaglandins that coat and protect the stomach. NSAIDs also increase production of stomach acid in general, and because they themselves are acidic, they expose GI tissue to increased amounts of acid. These ulcerogenic effects can result in potentially lethal GI bleeding in the setting of NSAID-induced platelet dysfunction. This ulcerogenic process is often silent due to the analgesic property of NSAID drugs.

are selected based on the degree of inflammation to be suppressed and tolerability. Acetaminophen (e.g., Tylenol), differs from other NSAIDs by blocking chemicals in peripheral nerves, rather than inflamed tissue. It does not affect platelet function and rarely causes GI distress, ulcers, or skin problems and is considered safer and better tolerated. The extent of renal or cardiovascular toxicity with long-term use of acetaminophen is currently being investigated. Acetaminophen, also referred to by its chemical name N-*a*cetyl-*p*ara-*a*mino*p*henol (APAP), will not interfere with skin or bone healing. Hepatotoxicity does occur with high doses or long-term use resulting in APAP being designated as the most common cause of drug-induced liver failure [22].

ALERT

Liver failure and acetaminophen: a dosage of 6 grams of APAP daily for 10 days will cause measurable liver damage. Young, healthy people should limit their APAP consumption to less than 4 g per day to prevent cumulative damage to the liver and kidneys. Elderly individuals and those with alcoholism, dehydration, or liver disease, should limit their APAP consumption to 2 g per day. Since the combination of alcohol and APAP accelerates liver damage, people should restrict APAP consumption to no more than 2 g on days when alcohol is consumed. A hidden ingredient in many over-the-counter (OTC) remedies, patients must be instructed to read the ingredient list of all OTC medicines they take to identify APAP.

Safety Precautions for NSAIDs

NSAIDs provide effective relief of pain and discomforts that result from trauma or inflammation. NSAIDs are an important drug class for mild, aching, and inflammatory pain, and are a fundamental component of multimodal therapy. The nurse should take a few safety precautions to prevent GI bleeding or other potentially harmful effects, including:

- Use the lowest effective dose for the shortest duration possible
- Have patient drink a full glass of water after swallowing the pill (unless fluid restricted)
- Take NSAIDs with food to reduce GI upset
- Remain upright for 20 to 30 min to minimize risk of esophageal irritation
- If taken regularly for more than 10 days, additional precautions are warranted
  - GI protection with a PPI, such as Prilosec OTC
  - Periodic monitoring of blood pressure, kidney, and liver functioning
  - Periodic testing for hidden GI bleeding and/or anemia

For patients at high risk (those with a past history of ulcers), the use of celecoxib with a PPI is considered. Patients who are taking aspirin for cardioprotective purposes need special consideration. Some NSAIDs, such as ibuprofen, inhibit the cardioprotective actions of aspirin, whereas others, such as naproxen, do not. Concurrent use of aspirin or other NSAIDs will undermine any gastroprotective advantage of celecoxib, whose gastroprotective advantage seems to wane after a year of ongoing therapy.

Opioid Analgesics

Opioids are medications that are chemically similar to opium that bind to and activate opioid receptors in the central nervous system (CNS) to block the transmission of pain signals. Opioid medications have variable effects on different subtypes of receptors (see Table 6–2). The prototype morphine, primarily binds with mu receptors, while a weak, partial agonist such as butorphanol (Stadol) activates kappa receptors. Most opioids also are classified as narcotics due to their habit-forming nature. The opioids vary in their abuse potential, and are classified accordingly by their "schedule" (see Table 6–3), which determines restriction of their prescription, storage, distribution, and use.

Weak or Mixed Opioids

The type of analgesic, previously referred to as Step 2 of the WHO analgesic ladder, includes

- Weak opioids
- Mixed opioids
  - Partial agonists
  - Mixed agonist-antagonists
  - Opioid, nonopioid compounds

 ON THE HORIZON

Topical NSAIDs are available with diclofenac gels and patches now commercially available and compounded ketoprofen is becoming more widely used. IV forms of COX-2 drugs and APAP, and Xefo (an NSAID with potency comparable with morphine) are used abroad but are not yet FDA approved. IV ibuprofen is becoming available for in-hospital use. Researchers are studying new drugs called p38 inhibitors that block COX-2 and other proinflammatory cytokines, such as tumor necrosis factor and interleukins. These are promising pain relievers that have fewer side effects than current options.

Table 6–2 Major Opioid Receptor Subtypes*

RECEPTOR TYPE	ACTION	COMMENT
Delta	Relieves pain Improves mood Contributes to development of physical dependence	Acts on the brain. Euphoric effects may contribute to abuse potential. Enkephalin-specific.
Kappa	Relieves pain Produces sedation and miosis (pupil constriction) Reduces GI motility Some hormonal (ADH) affects, diuresis Produces some psychotomimetic effects (hallucinations), and dysphoria	Acts on the brain and spine. Butorphanol (Stadol) used clinically; significantly selective; naloxone antagonistic at all three sites. Dynorphin-specific.
Mu	Relieves pain Depresses respirations Produces sedation and miosis Improves mood, possibly to the state of euphoria Contributes to development of physical dependence Reduces GI motility	Acts on brain and spine. Site of action for morphine, fentanyl, and other pure opioid antagonists. naloxone and naltrexone act antagonistically. Endorphin-specific.
ORL-1 Opioid-receptorlike 1	Unclear role in pain relief No sedation or respiratory depression Nociceptin or orphanin activate the receptor and influence the intensity of pain signals.	Recently discovered opioid receptor. Once understood better, drugs to target or block its effect may be developed.

*Opioid receptors are specific sites on the cell surface that interact in a highly selective fashion with both endogenous (e.g., endorphins) or exogenous (medications) opioids. Different opioid medications activate and/or block one or more of these receptors to produce their clinical effect. A better understanding of these receptors and their subtypes is helping scientists design more effective pain relievers with a lower side effect burden.

Useful for moderate pain, weak and mixed opioids are generally 2 to 4 times more potent than nonopioids alone, although they share the risks of both drug classes. These drugs have a ceiling effect and a narrower therapeutic index than pure opioids.

Table 6–3 Controlled Substances in the United States

CLASS	COMMENTS
Schedule I (C-I)	Highest abuse potential. No approved medical use. Examples: marijuana, heroin, LSD
Schedule II (C-II)	High-abuse potential. Medically necessary drugs that produce physical or psychological dependence. Prescriptions can be written, but may not be transmitted by phone or refilled. Restrictions on the number of units (pills) that can be dispensed per prescription exist and may vary by state. Examples: morphine, oxycodone, meperidine, fentanyl, oxymorphone, methadone, parenteral codeine. Nonanalgesic examples: cocaine, methylphenidate
Schedule III (C-III)	Abuse potential is lower than Schedule I-II. Moderate/low risk of physical dependence. Moderate/high risk of psychological dependence. Legitimate, medically necessary drugs. Telephone orders and limited refills are acceptable. Examples: Hydrocodone, codeine, dihydrocodeine pills combined with acetaminophen, buprenorphine Nonanalgesic examples: Anabolic steroids, paregoric.
Schedule IV (C-IV)	Abuse potential lower than Schedule I-III. Low risk of physical or psychological dependence or abuse. Legitimate, medically necessary uses. Telephone orders and limited refills acceptable. Examples: Butorphanol, propoxyphene Nonanalgesic examples: Alprazolam, midazolam, phenobarbitol
Schedule V (C-V)	Lowest abuse potential. Low risk of physical/psychological dependence. Legitimate, medically necessary uses. Telephone orders & refills ok. Limited amounts can be made available to adults without prescription (cough). Examples: Tylenol with codeine elixir, codeine-containing cough preparations; diphenoxylate, opium preparations
Noteworthy exception	Tramadol (e.g., Ultram), a weak opioid agonist that has norepinephrine and serotonin reuptake inhibition actions; believed to have lower abuse potential than other opioids, is available by prescription but it is not scheduled.

Weak Opioids

The weak opioids are codeine, tramadol, and propoxyphene. Therapeutic doses of these medicines are only slightly more potent than aspirin; thus they tend to be useful only when mixed with other analgesics (i.e., aspirin or acetaminophen). Propoxyphene (e.g., Darvocet), is no stronger than aspirin and has many safety and toxicity problems, especially when used in older adults. Even at typical therapeutic doses, weak opioids can have serious side effects, including:

- Codeine has problematic GI side effects
- Propoxyphene produces a byproduct that irritates the heart, nerves, and muscles
- Tramadol can result in seizures at high doses

Codeine may be a good option for some people who metabolize it properly, but many people lack the enzyme required to convert it to the active (morphine) form, and others metabolize it in an ultrarapid way and get an exaggerated response. Among the weak opioids, tramadol may have an advantage for chronic pain, because it is non-narcotic and has desirable effects on serotonin and norepinephrine reuptake in the spine.

Mixed Agonist-Antagonists

This group includes drugs that bind to some opioid receptors while blocking others. Buprenorphine (parenteral Buprenex or sublingual Suboxone) partially activates mu receptors while blocking the kappa receptors. In contrast, other agonist-antagonist drugs, such as pentazocine (Talwin), butorphanol (Stadol), or nalbuphine (Nubain) block mu receptors while activating kappa receptors. Some formulations add naloxone which will precipitate a withdrawal syndrome if an opioid dependent person tries to alter it for self-injection.

Buprenorphine has a high affinity for the mu receptors, but can only activate its analgesic effects partially. Buprenorphine also blocks kappa receptors (associated with sedation, pain relief, and euphoria) activity. This drug has good analgesic effect, while it blocks euphoria, and may produce dysphoric effects. A ceiling effect occurs to both the analgesic and respiratory depressant effects, so that increasing the dose beyond a certain point will fail to provide more relief, but will not increase the risk of slowing respirations. Because it binds so strongly at the mu receptor, once buprenorphine is given, morphine, heroin, and even naloxone cannot work. This makes buprenorphine an alternative to methadone for narcotic treatment programs. The safety and favorable side effect profile make it an increasingly popular analgesic choice.

The other mixed agonist-antagonist drugs relieve pain by activating kappa receptors while blocking mu receptors. Patients who have taken a pure opioid agonist for more than a week have developed some degree of physical dependence and may have a serious withdrawal reaction when exposed to these mixed drugs, even if used as directed. Therefore, mixed agonist-antagonists may be useful in select opioid-naïve patients with infrequent, single-dose use, but patients should not be switched from opioids to these preparations. Table 6–4 lists common examples of weak and mixed opioids.

Mixed Opioid, Nonopioid Combinations

The mixed opioids subgroup has a low-dose, strong opioid component combined with a nonopioid analgesic, such as APAP or ibuprofen. The nonopioid ingredient limits the amount of these medications a patient safely can take. For example, the combination oxycodone-APAP preparations, such as

Table 6–4 Examples of Weak or Mixed Opioids

GENERIC NAME & BRAND EXAMPLES	ANALGESIC DOSE (ADULT)	DOSING INTERVAL	ROUTE(S)	COMMENTS
MIXED OPIOIDS				
Oxycodone combined with aspirin, APAP, or ibuprofen (Percocet, Combunox)	5–10 mg	every 4 or every 6 hr	Oral	Nonopioid component is dose-limiting. Without the additive, oxycodone is a strong opioid with high doses possible.
Hydrocodone 5-, 7.5-, or 10-mg strengths (Vicodin, Lortab, Norco, Zydone)	5–10 mg	every 4 or every 6 hr	Oral	Available in combination products. Nonopioid component is dose-limiting (e.g., limit APAP=<2–4 g/day)
WEAK OPIOIDS				
Tramadol (Ultram, Ultracet)	50–100 mg (≤400 mg/day)	every 4 or every 6 hr	Oral	A weak opioid also blocks serotonin & norepinephrine reuptake. Serious side effects are uncommon.

Continued

Table 6–4 Examples of Weak or Mixed Opioids—cont'd

GENERIC NAME & BRAND EXAMPLES	ANALGESIC DOSE (ADULT)	DOSING INTERVAL	ROUTE(S)	COMMENTS
WEAK OPIOIDS (cont'd)				
Propoxyphene napsylate (Balacet, Darvon-N compound, Darvocet-N)	65 mg	every 4 or every 6 hr	Oral	65 mg propoxyphene is no stronger than aspirin. Compounds tend to have very high APAP doses. Propoxyphene metabolizes to norpropoxyphene, which is toxic to nerve and cardiac tissue.
Codeine (Tylenol 3, Empirin 3)	30–60 mg	every 4 or every 6 hr	Oral (injection available but rarely used)	30 mg oral codeine is equipotent with 325 mg APAP. 10% of the population lacks the enzyme to convert codeine to morphine. Ceiling effect at and dose limiting side effects > 60 mg.
AGONIST-ANTAGONIST				
Butorphanol (Stadol)	2–3 mg	every 4 hr	Parenteral or intranasal	Kappa receptor agonist, mu antagonist. Can precipitate withdrawal in opioid-dependent patients. Nasal spray useful for migraines.
Pentazocine (Talwin)	50 mg PO 30 mg IV, IM, or SQ	every 3 or every 4 hr	Oral or parenteral	Kappa receptor agonist, mu antagonist. Can precipitate withdrawal in opioid-dependent patients.

Percocet contain 325 mg acetaminophen per tablet. In otherwise healthy patients to stay below the 4-g limit, daily use is limited to 12 tablets. In contrast, the hydrocodone-APAP combination Vicodin ES, each pill contains 750 mg of acetaminophen. Persons who are elderly, dehydrated, or have any liver disorders need to restrict intake of this product to no more than 2 and one-half tablets to stay below the daily 2-g APAP limit.

Strong Opioids

Strong opioids, also known as pure opioid agonist analgesics, include opium derivatives (e.g., morphine) and synthetic analogs (e.g., fentanyl or methadone) [4]. Pure agonists relieve pain primarily by binding to opiate receptors in the spine and brain. Among a variety of receptor-types, the mu receptors found in peripheral and central nerves; and CNS-based kappa opioid receptors, are believed to have important roles in pain control. Analgesia is believed to result from diminished presynaptic Ca^{++} influx, which lowers the production and release of chemical messengers of pain and alters sodium permeability. On the postsynaptic membrane, activation of the opioid receptors lowers nerve excitability following enhanced K^+ movement out of the cells. Opioids also act peripherally on inflamed tissue to lower the transduction of pain signals. These drugs are the most potent class of pain relievers, and are medically necessary for severe pain or when other medications have failed to control moderate pain.

> **ALERT**
>
> Avoid drugs with toxic metabolites. Meperidine (Demerol) is avoided because of its short half-life and accumulating metabolite (normeperidine), which can induce seizures. Meperidine relieves pain for 3 hr, but the half-life of toxic normeperidine is close to 30 hr. At doses of 600 mg per day, or when used for more than 48 hr, the risk of neurotoxicity and seizures is high. Similarly, the toxic metabolite of propoxyphene (Darvon) accumulates (half-life > 30 hr) often producing psychological disturbances and cardiac arrhythmias.

 NURSE-TO-NURSE TIP

Estimated dosages for an opioid-tolerant patient can be based on the patient's known responses to a specific medication. For opioid-naïve patients, there is not a precise standard dose that is safe and effective. Significant individual variability in drug metabolizing enzymes, nerve structure and function, degree of pain, and concurrent drugs or diseases make it difficult to predict responses. Start an opioid-naïve patient at what is considered a safe initial dose for his or her pain level (Table 6–5), monitor the patient's response, and adjust the dose or interval accordingly.

Table 6–5	Suggested Starting Oral Doses for Opioid-Naïve Patients*			
MEDICATION	ORAL	PARENTERAL	DOSE FREQUENCY
OPIOID-NONOPIOID COMPOUND (*MODERATE* PAIN)			
Codeine	30–60 mg	N/A	q 3 or 4 hr
Hydrocodone (e.g., Lorcet, Lortab, Vicodin)	5–10 mg	N/A	q 3 or 4 hr
Oxycodone (e.g., Roxicodone, Percocet, Tylox, Norco)	5 mg	N/A	q 3 or 4 hr
OPIOID AGONIST (*SEVERE* PAIN)			
Morphine	10–20 mg	2–5 mg	q 3 or 4 hr
Hydromorphone (Dilaudid)	4–8 mg	0.5–1 mg	q 3 or 4 hr
Oxycodone	5–15 mg	N/A	q 3 or 4 hr

*These doses are conservative and not equipotent. Further reductions may be needed for elderly patients of for those with renal or hepatic insufficiency.

Pharmacovigilance

When administering any analgesic, the nurse must vigilantly prevent medication errors and monitor patients for the development of adverse effects. Common opioid errors to avoid are:

- Improper drug selection (e.g., using fentanyl or methadone for opioid-naïve patients)
- Improper patient selection (e.g., patient-controlled analgesia for unconscious patients)
- Name confusion (look-alike, sound-alike drugs) resulting in a wrong drug error
- Dosage errors (e.g., substituting mg for mL, or selecting a wrong concentration)*

---

* Opioids should be ordered by dose (mg) rather than volume (mL). The Joint Commission and the Institute for Safe Medication Practices suggest the abbreviation "mL" be used instead of "cc" to designate volume. See http://www.ismp.org/Tools/errorproneabbreviations.pdf or http://www. jointcommission.org/patientsafety/donotuselist/

- Incorrect route of administration (e.g., tube confusion, IV versus epidural)
- Improper timing of drug administration (especially accumulating drugs, such as fentanyl)
- Improper alteration of the drug (e.g., cutting an OxyContin tablet or fentanyl patch)

Adverse Effects of Opioids

Additionally, nurses must observe for adverse effects of opioids. Sedation, nausea, vomiting, urinary retention, and respiratory depression may be noted initially. With long-term use, sexual dysfunction, and constipation are common. The most serious adverse effect is respiratory depression (≤ 8 respirations per min), which usually occurs early in therapy among opioid naive patients or during authorized or unauthorized dose escalation. Serious respiratory depression also can occur as a result of drug-drug or drug-disease interactions. Clinically, the patient will appear overly sedated, respirations will progressively slow and deepen, and periods of apnea will occur. Box 6–2 shows an example of a sedation scale typically used to monitor patients on opioids.

Tolerance to Adverse Effects

Patients generally develop tolerance to the sedative and respiratory-depressant effects of opioids after a few days of therapy. For patients who require ongoing opioid therapy, tolerance develops to the nauseating and

---

Box 6–2 Pasero Opioid-Induced Sedation Scale (POSS)*

S = Sleep, easy to arouse
1 = Awake & alert
2 = Slightly drowsy, easily aroused
3 = Frequently drowsy, arousable, drifts off to sleep during conversation
4 = Somnolent, minimal, or no response to physical stimulation

*POSS is copyright of Chris Pasero, 1994. Reprinted with permission.

emetic effects after 1 or 2 weeks . Unfortunately, tolerance to the constipating or hormone-suppressing effects does not occur. Table 6–6 lists suggested measures to prevent and treat side effects of opioid analgesics.

Tolerance to Pain-Relieving Effects

Tolerance to the pain-relieving effects of opioids may occur through a variety of mechanisms, including:

- Hepatic enzyme induction (increases rate of opioid metabolism)
- Toxic metabolite accumulation (may excite pain fibers)
- Interneuronal enzyme changes (increase nerve excitability)
- Reduced production and release of endorphins (natural morphinelike chemicals)
- Reduced number of opioid receptors at the synapse
- N-methyl-D-aspartate (NMDA)-receptor activation (produces a hyperalgesic and neurotoxic state)

These associated neurological changes can account, for **opioid-induced hyperalgesia.** This phenomenon occurs when opioid-tolerant patients become more sensitive to pain or develop new areas of pain; in addition to a loss of the drug's original potency. Awareness of this phenomenon has stimulated much debate and research into the best ways to treat patients on long-term opioids. One strategy is to limit the dose and duration of therapy, another is to switch patients to a different opioid. Methadone has been a popular choice, because many people do not develop tolerance to it. Given methadone's apparent ability to undo some of these mechanisms of tolerance, overdose can occur during the switching process if prudent dose-reduction steps (described below) are not followed.

Opioid Equianalgesia

The term **equianalgesia** refers to the relative potency of different opioid analgesics. Typically morphine is the reference drug, and **morphine**

Table 6-6 Management of Common Opioid Side Effects

SIDE EFFECT	COMMENTS
Constipation	Start bowel regimen along with opioid: begin with stool softener and a mild stimulant laxative, such as Senokot-S. Methylnaltrexone bromide (SQ injection is used in the most severe cases when all else fails).
Sedation	Tolerance may develop. Reduce dose or switch opioids. Reduce use of other CNS depressants. Check respirations. May try CNS stimulant (methylphenidate) or modafinil.
Bradypnea/apnea	Stimulate and prompt to breathe. Interrupt opioid exposure. Administer narcan slowly if unresponsive and respirations ≤8/min. May need to follow with a Narcan infusion until opioid wears off.
Nausea/vomiting	Tolerance may develop. Try prochlorperazine or ondansetron. Reduce dose or switch opioid.
Pruritus	Reduce dose or switch opioid. Consider diphenhydramine (and associated risk of sedation).
Mental change (e.g., delirium)	Reduce dose or switch opioid. Consider haloperidol or risperidone.

equivalents are used to compare the potency of other drugs to that of parenteral morphine. The equianalgesic chart (Table 6–7) and equianalgesic calculators are tools to help professionals estimate safe starting doses, guide the adjustment of medications, or switch from one drug or route of administration to another in a safe and effective manner. Dose conversion calculators, such as http://www.globalrph.com/narcoticonv.htm, are available online. The two manual calculating techniques used to determine safe, effective starting doses using equianalgesic equivalents are the ratio and cross-multiplication methods.

The Ratio Technique

The **ratio technique** involves calculating the equipotency dose based on the proportionate strength of the current agent or route.

Switching Routes

For example, when changing the route of administration of morphine, Table 6–7 shows that the parenteral (IV) route is 3 times more potent than

Table 6–7 Equianalgesic Chart*

DRUG	PARENTERAL DOSE	ORAL DOSE	COMMENTS
Morphine	10 mg	30 mg	Higher oral to IV dose ratios (6:1) may be needed early in therapy.
Meperidine	75 mg	300 mg	Avoid use due to toxic effects.
Fentanyl	0.1 mg (100 mcg)	100 mcg (buccal)	Buccal formulations only for breakthrough pain in opioid–tolerant patients.
Dilaudid (HYDRO-morPHONE)	1.5 mg	7.5 mg	The brand name and special TALLman lettering is used because hydroMORPHone is the most common drug cited in sound-alike, look-alike (wrong drug) errors.
Hydrocodone	NA	20 mg	Nonopioid ingredient limits dose.
Codeine	130 mg	200 mg	Doses listed are higher than the analgesic ceiling and maximum tolerated dose of 60 mg for most patients.
Oxymorphone	1 mg	10 mg	This drug may be more potent in older adults or when taken with food or alcohol.
Oxycodone	NA	20 mg	Available in combination products and as a single agent (both Immediate Release or Sustained Release), enhancing its utility.
Methadone	10 mg	20 mg	These values may be used for a switch *from Methadone* to another agent. When switching from another agent *TO Methadone* use the ratios below.

Continued

Table 6–7 Equianalgesic Chart*—cont'd

EQUIANALGESIC CONVERSION TO ORAL METHADONE		
Oral Morphine Equivalent	Mg of oral = Mg of oral Methadone (ratio) Morphine	
<100 mg/day	1	4
101–300 mg/day	1	8
301– 600 mg/day	1	10
601–800 mg/day	1	12
801–1,000 mg/day	1	15
> 1,000 mg/day	1	20

*Ayonrinde OT, Bridge DT. (2000). The rediscovery of methadone for cancer pain management. *Medical Journal of Australia, 173*:536-540.

the oral route. The oral-to-IV morphine ratio is 3:1. As such, a patient on an IV morphine drip running at a rate of 4 mg/hr is receiving nearly 100 mg IV morphine per day and will require 300 mg of *oral* morphine per day to control the same level of pain. This analgesic need can be met with 150 mg of sustained-release oral morphine every 12 hr *or* 50 mg of immediate-release oral morphine every 4 hr.

Similarly, parenteral hydromorphone (Dilaudid) has 5 times the potency of oral preparations (oral:IV ratio of 5:1). A patient who requires 30 mg of oral Dilaudid per day (5 mg every 4 hr) would need only 6 mg of IV Dilaudid per day (0.25 mg per hr) to achieve the same level of analgesia.

Switching Medications

When a patient has required multiple dose escalations over a period of weeks or months, it is assumed that some degree of tolerance to that agent has occurred. When switching from one opioid to another, an additional step is added to account for limited cross-tolerance between agents; the calculated dose is reduced by 25% to 50%. For example:

- 10 mg of *IV* morphine = 10 mg of *oral* oxymorphone (1:1 ratio)
- A patient on a morphine drip (for 10 days) needs 2 mg per hr (48 mg IV morphine/day)
- 48 mg *IV* morphine per day = 48 mg *oral* oxymorphone per day
- Recommended starting dose is 24 to 36 mg/day (25% to 50% reduction) *oral* oxymorphone
  - 25% reduction if pain *is not* well controlled on current regimen
  - 50% reduction if pain *is* well controlled, with intolerable side effects on the current regimen
  - Consider how the new medication is supplied and determine a reasonable starting dose (e.g., 30 mg/day), either
    - 15 mg Opana ER (extended release) every 12 hr–*OR*
    - 5 mg Opana every 4 hr
- Carefully monitor patient's response and adjust as needed after switching

The Cross-Multiplication Technique

Another calculation method involves a **cross-multiplication technique** (different correct methods exist). A fraction is set up with the numerator representing the equianalgesia chart value of the current medication and the denominator representing the equivalent amount of the desired medication as listed on the chart (this fraction = 1 because of their presumed equipotence). On the other side of the equation the current dose of the medication in use is listed over X (the amount to be calculated) of the desired medication. Cross-multiplication is used to solve for X.

Consider the hypothetical case of Jane, a cervical cancer patient whose pain has been satisfactorily controlled with a stable dose of oral morphine for several months, but who has developed hyperalgesia and myoclonus, believed to be secondary to the morphine (after other causes have been ruled out). A switch to oral oxycodone is indicated. Currently, she is taking 45 mg of sustained release oral morphine (MS-SR) every 12 hr, plus 10 mg of immediate release oral morphine (MS-IR) used consistently at least 3 times daily for breakthrough pain. Jane can be established on a long-acting opioid to meet her anticipated daily requirement. Provisions for doses of a short-acting opioid should be made available for episodic (breakthrough) pain, and prophylactically for anticipated (dressing change, procedural) pain. Typically, these short-term doses consist of 10% to 20% of the total 24-hr dose and are made available every 2 hr prn. See Figure 6–2.

Switching Opioids: Oral Morphine to Oral Oxycodone

Jane takes 45 mg oral morphine sulfate-SR every 12 hours; plus 10 mg of morphine sulfate -IR 3 times a day. A calculation to determine an equivalent amount of oxycodone is based on actual morphine use.

Step 1: Determine the total current 24-hour opioid requirement:

Sustained release (MS-SR):   45 mg x 2   = 90 mg/24 hrs
Short-acting (MS-IR):   10 mg x 3   = 30 mg/24 hrs
            90 + 30 = 120 mg of oral morphine per day

Step 2: Set up an equianalgesic equation:

Equianalgesic Doses	
Oral (mg)	**Drug**
30	Morphine
20	Oxycodone

$$\frac{\text{Equianalgesic Table dose of current drug}}{\text{Equianalgesic Table dose of new drug}} = \frac{24° \text{ dose current drug}}{X \ (24° \text{ dose new drug})}$$

$$\frac{30 \text{ mg oral morphine}}{20 \text{ mg oral oxycodone}} = \frac{120 \text{ mg/day morphine}}{X \text{ mg/day oxycodone}}$$

Step 3: Solve for **X**: $\dfrac{30 \text{ mg oral morphine}}{20 \text{ mg oral oxycodone}}$ $\dfrac{120 \text{ mg/day morphine}}{X \text{ mg/day oxycodone}}$

a) 30**X** = 120 x 20
b) **X** = 2400/30
c) **X** = 80 mg

Solving for **X** = 2400/30 = 80 mg oxycodone q 24 hours

Step 4: Decrease by 50% for incomplete cross-tolerance.
     80 x 0.5 = 40 mg total 24-hour dose

Step 5: Divide by the number of doses per day. Oxycodone SR 40 mg per day in 2 doses.
     40 mg /day in 2 doses = 20 mg q12 hours

Step 6: Add prn rescue dosing 10%–20% daily dose (4–8 mg oral oxycodone) available q 2 hours

Thus the calculated safe, effective starting point for Jane is:

Oxycodone SR (OxyContin) 20 mg q12 hours
Oxycodone IR 2.5–5 mg q 2 hours prn breakthrough pain

Step 7: Monitor patient closely for balance of analgesia, function, and side effects

Step 8: In 24 hours review total dose received, effect, and recalculate scheduled dose as indicated

F I G U R E 6 – 2 : Switching opioids: oral morphine to oral oxycodone (Jane).

The transcription fentanyl patch and methadone are two noteworthy exceptions to this method of calculation. Both are drugs that accumulate and require careful monitoring over a period of several days before the transition is complete. Both also require the professional to convert the patient's current opioid requirement into oral morphine equivalents.

Switching to Transdermal Fentanyl

The manufacturer of transdermal fentanyl provides a dose guide in the package insert (see the first and last columns on Table 6–8). The remaining columns in Table 6–8 will help the reader approximate the doses of common analgesics in the middle of the suggested range. The estimates given are conservative, partly because the manufacturer has already built in a 50% dose reduction, so no further dose reduction is needed.

ALERT

Methadone is an excellent analgesic, is stable with long-term therapy and is inexpensive. However, its unique properties (long and variable half-life of 8 to 90 hr), potential cardiac effects, and drug-drug interactions make converting to methadone complex. Rapid dose titration early in therapy has led to serious respiratory depression, even death. Therefore patients need close monitoring during the initial titration phase (first week of therapy) and any time the dose is escalated.

The onset of action for transdermal fentanyl is variable (12 to 24 hr), with the peak action expected between 18 and 30 hr after the patch is applied. Therefore, an overlap period of approximately 12 hr with the previous opioid is required, but double dosing during the second 12 hr must be avoided. With subsequent patch applications, the old patch must be removed completely before the new patch is applied. Situations causing the area of the patch to be heated (i.e., fever, sunbathing, hot tub, heating pad, MRI) must be avoided to prevent overdose from enhanced absorption.

Switching to Methadone

Methadone also has its own conversion procedure. Use of methadone use for analgesia has increased in recent years because it is inexpensive, can be dosed 3 or 4 times daily, is safe to use during pregnancy and lactation, and seems to counter the effects of tolerance. Thus many people do not experience increased dose requirements over time. One potential problem is the remote risk of a deadly cardiac irregularity (torsade de pointes) that can occur at any dose but is seen most often at dosages more than 100 mg/day. Another concern is the additional steps required to calculate a safe starting dose when switching an opioid tolerant patient to methadone, such as that described in the case of John (see Fig. 6–3). Once a patient is switched to methadone, dose escalations are avoided for several days until the patient achieves steady state.

Table 6-8 Fentanyl Transdermal (TD) Patch Equianalgesic Conversion*

TRANSDERMAL FENTANYL (MCG/HR)	PARENTERAL MORPHINE EQUIVALENT (MG/HR) TO TD FENTANYL	PARENTERAL (DILAUDID) EQUIVALENT (MG/HR) TO TD FENTANYL	ORAL OXYCODONE EQUIVALENT (MG/DAY) TO TD FENTANYL	MANUFACTURER'S RANGE FOR ORAL MORPHINE EQUIVALENT (MG/DAY) TO TD FENTANYL	APS GUIDE TO POTENCY CONVERSIONS FROM ORAL MORPHINE (MG/DAY) TO TD FENTANYL
12**mcg/hr	0.3 mg/hr	0.05 mg/hr	20 mg/day	60-134 mg/day	30-90 mg/day
25***mcg/hr	0.6 mg/hr	0.1 mg/hr	45 mg/day	135-224 mg/day	91-150 mg/day
50**mcg/hr	1.3 mg/hr	0.2 mg/hr	90 mg/day	225-314 mg/day	151-210 mg/day
75**mcg/hr	1.8 mg/hr	0.3 mg/hr	135 mg/day	315-404 mg/day	211-270 mg/day
100**mcg/hr	2.5 mg/hr	0.4 mg/hr	180 mg/day	405-494 mg/day	271-330 mg/day
125 mcg/hr	3.1 mg/hr	0.5 mg/hr	225 mg/day	495-584 mg/day	331-390 mg/day
150 mcg/hr	3.7 mg/hr	0.6 mg/hr	270 mg/day	585-674 mg/day	391-450 mg/day
175 mcg/hr	4.3 mg/hr	0.7 mg/hr	315 mg/day	675-764 mg/day	451-510 mg/day
200 mcg/hr	5 mg/hr	0.8 mg/hr	360 mg/day	765-854 mg/day	511-570 mg/day
225 mcg/hr	5.5 mg/hr	0.8 mg/hr	400 mg/day	855-944 mg/day	571-630 mg/day
250 mcg/hr	6.3 mg/hr	0.9 mg/hr	450 mg/day	945-1,034 mg/day	631-690 mg/day
275 mcg/hr	6.8 mg/hr	1 mg/hr	500 mg/day	945-1,034 mg/day	631-690 mg/day
300 mcg/hr	7.4 mg/hr	1.1 mg/hr	540 mg/day	1035-1,124 mg/day	691-750 mg/day

*NOTE: Doses listed here are approximately at the midpoint of the range provided by the manufacturer. The manufacturer bases the conversion to TD Fentanyl on conservative estimates compared to those of the American Pain Society (APS) analgesic guidelines (2008).
** Commercially available patch sizes. NOTE: 12 mcg/hr patch delivers 12.5 mcg/hr, however "12 label" minimizes "wrong dose" (125 mcg/hr) errors.

Switching Opioids: Oral Oxycodone to IV Methadone

John is 48 with metastatic esophageal cancer on escalating doses of oxycodone-ER for 6 months. Current dose is 280 mg OxyContin PO q8h plus oxycodone-IR 5 mg PO q4h prn (4 doses /day)

Step 1: Determine the total current 24-hour opioid requirement of current medication:

Extended release (Oxycodone-ER):	280 mg x 3	= 840 mg/24 hrs
Short-acting (Oxycodone-IR):	5 mg x 4	= +20 mg/24 hrs
	840 + 20	= 860 mg oxycodone/day

Step 2: Set up an equianalgesic equation to determine oral morphine equivalent:

$$\frac{\text{Equianalgesic Table dose of current drug}}{\text{Equianalgesic Table dose of new drug}} = \frac{24° \text{ dose current drug}}{\textbf{X} \ (24° \text{ dose new drug})}$$

$$\frac{20 \text{ mg oral oxycodone}}{30 \text{ mg oral morphine}} = \frac{860 \text{ mg/day oxycodone}}{\textbf{X} \text{ mg/day oral morphine}}$$

Step 3: Solve for **X**:

$$\frac{20 \text{ mg oral oxycodone}}{30 \text{ mg oral morphine}} \diagdown\diagup \frac{860 \text{ mg/day oxycodone}}{\textbf{X} \text{ mg/day oral morphine}}$$

a) 860 x 30 = 20**X**
b) 25,800/20 = **X**
c) 1290 mg = **X**

Thus John requires 1290 mg of oral morphine equivalents per day to control his cancer pain

Step 4: Calculate starting dose of oral methadone for a patient using over 1000 mg of oral morphine per day. A 20:1 ratio is used.* 1290 mg/20 = 64.5 mg of oral methadone.

Step 5: Decrease starting dose by 50% to account for incomplete cross-tolerance.
64.5 mg X 0.5 = 32.25 mg of oral methadone per day

Step 6: Divide dose by 50% as IV methadone is about twice the potency of oral methadone: 32 x 0.5 = 16 mg IV methadone

Step 7: Calculate intermittent dose or continuous rate.

16 mg/day given in 4 divided doses would be 4 mg Methadone IV q 6 hours
-or-
16 mg/day given in a continuous IV drip (16/24) would start at 0.7 mg/hour

*See Table 6-7

F I G U R E 6 – 3 : Switching opioids: oral oxycodone to IV methadone (John).

Administering and Evaluating the Effects of Opioids

All opioids are high-alert medications demanding that nurses take steps to prevent medication errors and remain vigilant in monitoring for medication, technology, or route-specific problems. Taking an extra moment to double-check the accuracy of orders and administration procedures can prevent serious side effects and accidental death. Nurses are urged to know and follow their organizations' procedures regarding high-alert medication precautions, preventing look-alike, sound-alike medication errors, and policies regarding double checks.

Opioids are most effective when given on schedule. Even those ordered on a prn basis should be offered when they are due, rather than waiting for the patient to ask. Within 1 hr after administering an opioid, reassess the patient for the extent of pain reduction, functional improvement, and presence or absence of adverse reactions.

Titrating Oral Opioids (Slow Method)

When the administered dose is ineffective, opioid doses are titrated to achieve the desired level of relief. The American Pain Society (2005) has developed algorithms for treating cancer pain based on route and the speed desired to control the pain. Their approach to slowly titrating *oral* opioids [23] is as follows.

- For opioid-naïve patients, start with 5 to 10 mg of short-acting oral morphine (or equivalent)
- For opioid-tolerant patients, start with a dose that is 25% to 50% higher than the patient's usual dose
- Reassess at 1 hr and readminister a dose in 4 hr based on the following:
  - The next dose is 25% to 50% higher if the pain is reduced by less that 50%
  - Repeat the same dose if pain is reduced by more than 50%, without limiting side effects

 NURSE-TO-NURSE TIP

Given individual response variability, opioids often are prescribed as range orders. Determining the best dose for a patient is based on factors other than the pain score alone. Generally opioid-naïve patients (especially elderly patients) are started with the lowest dose in the prescribed range and observed for effect. Prior response to opioids (analgesia and side effects), recovery trajectory, comorbidities, other medications, psychosocial factors, and environmental factors are all part of nursing judgment of the best dose to administer.

- Reassess in 1 hr and repeat the cycle every 4 hr
- Reassess the patient 24 to 48 hr after starting the process
  - If pain intensity remains < 4 (on a 0-10 scale), convert to a scheduled long-action opioid based on the previous day's total dose
- Make 10% to 20% of daily dose available q 2 hr prn for breakthrough pain
  - If pain remains high (> 5/10) continue to titrate as above (increasing the dose by 25% to 50%) until pain is controlled for 24 hr before converting to a long-acting opioid
  - Monitor, manage side effects, and educate the patient and family

Titrating IV Opioids (Rapid Method)

Given the perspective that uncontrolled severe pain is a crisis situation, much like a code [24], there also is a *rapid IV method* of controlling pain [24]:

- For opioid-naïve patients, start with 2 to 5 mg IV morphine (or equivalent)
- For opioid-tolerant patients, start with an IV dose equal to 10% to 20% of the patient's usual daily dose
- Reassess pain and respirations in 15 min then administer another dose at that time if respiratory rate is adequate. Dose amount is determined by the following:
  - If pain is unchanged, administer double the prior dose and reassess in 15 min
  - If pain is reduced by less than 50%, repeat the prior dose and reassess in 15 min
- Repeat these steps every 15 min until the pain is cut by 50% or respirations are below 10
- Once pain is controlled, calculate the dose needed to be effective (either hourly or daily)
  - Administer the anticipated dose as needed in a drip or scheduled doses
  - Make additional medication doses available for breakthrough pain (BTP)
  - 10% to 20% of daily opioid amount available every 2 hr prn
  - Monitor, manage side effects, and educate the patient and family

Further adjustments up or down, may be needed over the next 1 or 2 days. Once the effective dose demonstrates a consistent pattern of relief, a schedule is established using long-acting opioids, (with supplemental short-acting drugs for BTP) to prevent analgesic gaps. After the first few days of titration, further adjustments are usually minimal unless there is a change in patient condition.

Tapering Schedules

Over time, the patient's analgesic requirement may wane, and a taper schedule may be used to avoid a withdrawal syndrome. The method of tapering varies depending on the drug used. A 10% to 25% reduction is generally safe with adjustments every 1 to 3 days for a short-acting opioid, and weekly adjustments for a long-acting opioid. Symptoms of withdrawal syndrome may still occur, and can be lessened with a clonidine transdermal (0.1 mg/24 hr) patch.

Patient Education

Patients and family members are educated about their particular analgesic regimen. This should include:

- Specific instructions for using the medication
- Signs and symptoms that must be reported to the doctor or nurse
- Importance of taking the medication only as prescribed
  - Only by the person it was prescribed for
  - Only for the reason it was prescribed for
  - Only in the manner it was prescribed
- Securing the medicine where others (e.g., children, visitors, etc.) cannot gain access to it
- Avoid alcohol
- Avoid taking other medications (including nonprescription medications and herbal products) unless authorized by the prescriber

Adjuvants Used for Pain Control

Adjuvant medications are not classified as pain medications, however they are components of the pain treatment plan. They may be selected with the goal to:

- Change certain features of the pain, such as
  - Less burning
  - Few bouts of sudden pain

 ON THE HORIZON

Investigational opioids hold promise for safer, more effective analgesia. Abuse-deterrent products designed to reduce the illicit use of prescription opioids are emerging. The active metabolite, morphine-6-glucuronide (M6G), is being refined to have the same potency of morphine with fewer side effects. New combination drugs and long-acting formulations of hydromorphone or nalbuphine are forthcoming. Genetically-engineered opioids that target specific receptor subtypes hold promise for better therapeutic options, especially for patients who need high-dose, long-term opioids.

- Less intense pain
- Less hyperalgesia or allodynia
- Relieve other discomforts that can worsen pain (spasm, insomnia, depression)
- Potentiate the effect of pain medications
- Reduce the pain medication's side effect burden

Pain-Altering Adjuvants

Examples of adjuvants that relieve pain are:

- Antidepressants (support the function of pain-modulating system)
- Anticonvulsants (stabilize nerve membranes, reducing excitability, and spontaneous firing)
- Local anesthetics (block the transmission of pain signals)

Relief of Other Discomforts

Anxiolytics, sedatives, and antispasmotics are examples of medicines that relieve other discomforts, but they do not alleviate pain and thus should be used in addition to, rather than instead of analgesics. Of note, when combined with opioids, sedatives increase the risk for respiratory depression and close monitoring is warranted.

Potentiating Effects

Some stimulants, such as caffeine or methamphetamine, are capable of potentiating the effect of other pain medications.

Reduction of Side Effects

Examples of medications used to reduce the side-effect burden of analgesics include antiemetics, laxatives, and stimulants.

Adjuvants for Neuropathic Pain

Adjuvants are particularly beneficial for the management of neuropathic pain (see Table 6–9). Tricyclic antidepressants (TCAs) are especially useful for central neuropathic pain and for diabetic neuropathy, which often manifests as pain with burning or unusual stinging qualities. The secondary amine TCAs (nortriptyline, desipramine) are preferred over the tertiary-amine TCAs (amitriptyline), due to a lower side-effect burden [17].

Selective serotonin and norepinephrine reuptake inhibitors (SNRIs), such as duloxetine, milnacipram, and venlafaxine, have a similar mechanism of

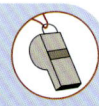

COACH CONSULT

Constipation is an almost universal adverse effect of opioid use. Patients should receive prophylactic stimulant laxative therapy, unless contraindicated. Stool softeners are not useful alone, but are a good choice when combined with a stimulant laxative (e.g., Senokot-S). If those products are ineffective, a regimen of cathartic laxatives (e.g., bisacodyl), followed by more aggressive treatment (i.e., osmotic laxatives, enema, manual disimpaction, and methylnaltrexone) may be necessary.

action as the TCAs, with an even lower side-effect burden. They also are considered first-line treatments for this type of pain.

Anticonvulsant drugs (gabapentin) are particularly useful for peripheral neuropathic conditions that often present with a stabbing, shooting, or electrical-shock quality. Local anesthetics, such as the Lidoderm patch

Table 6–9 Selected Adjuvant Drugs Useful for Neuropathic Pain

GENERIC NAME	ANALGESIC DOSE (ADULT START)	DOSING INTERVAL	ADEQUATE TRIAL	COMMENTS
Desipramine, nortriptyline (Norpramin, Pamelor)	10–25 mg	Daily at bedtime	Titrated to 100–150 mg for at least 2 weeks at maximum tolerated dose (6 weeks total)	Anticholinergic side effects may limit use. Helps sleep and mood. Use cautiously in patients with cardiac disease, glaucoma, seizure disorder, or who are taking other serotonin reuptake inhibitors.
Duloxetine (Cymbalta)	30 mg	Daily	60 mg once or twice daily for 4 weeks	Lower side-effect burden than TCA (desipramine).
Gabapentin (Neurontin)	100–300 mg	First dose hs, then tid	1,800–3,600 mg per day for 1 month at maximum tolerated dose	Sedation, dizziness, and edema are major dose-limiting effects. Improves sleep and anxiety. Routine liver test not needed; use caution with patients with renal disease.
Pregabalin (Lyrica)	50 mg	tid	600 mg per day for 4 weeks	Same as gabapentin. Generally better tolerated and easier to titrate than gabapentin.
Topical Lidocaine (5%) patch (Lidoderm)	1–3 patches (depends on pain area)	On 12–18 hr	Daily patches for 3 weeks	Local skin irritation because patch gets placed in the same location (on pain) every day.

There are many new pain-relieving drugs in the pipeline that do not fit into the class of NSAIDs or opioids. Some prevent the intensification of pain by inactivating specific sodium channels or blocking collapsin-response proteins. Others prevent neuroplastic changes that convert acute pain into chronic pain. Others target the amino acids, neuropeptides, neurotransmitters, and receptors known to transmit pain. Exciting developments in agents that are active on the NMDA-receptor hold promise not only to treat stubborn pain but also to prevent and treat tolerance or opioid-induced hyperalgesia.

alleviate neuropathic and other types of pain and are particularly useful for patients with the skin sensitivity known as allodynia.

In the event those medications do not work alone, in combination, or in conjunction with opioids, second- and third-line strategies are available [17]. Different anticonvulsant drugs (i.e., carbamazepine, valproic acid, lamotrigine, or oxcarbazepine), antidepressant drugs (i.e., citalopram, paroxetine, or bupropion) or mexiletine may be tried for those who fail first-line therapy. Occasionally topical capsaicin provides benefit. As a derivative of strong peppers, it is believed to lower the concentration of pain sensitizer Substance P. Many find the burning sensation and demanding application schedule problematic, but it is effective for some people. For patients with intrathecal analgesia devices in place, an N-type calcium channel blocker (ziconotide) is available for clinical use.

There are many new drug classes for pain in various stages of research development. Examples of new classes of drugs include:

- New nonopioids that block different anti-inflammatory targets (p38, tumor necrosis factor, interleukins)
- Genetically engineered opioids that target specific receptor subtypes
- Drugs that inactivate specific neurotransmitters, sodium channels, proteins, amino acids, and other receptors.
- NMDA blockers
- Drugs that block the upregulation, or hasten the downregulation of non-neuronal cells, such as the microglia

The rapid advancement in understanding the mechanisms of different pain types has stimulated scientific and clinical investigations that hold promise that better pain-relieving drugs will be available in the near future. While the search for the "perfect drug" continues, a multimodal approach with attention to the individualized details of safety and efficacy remains the best way to relieve pain.

7 Nondrug, Complementary, and Alternative Medicine Approaches to Pain Relief

CHAPTER 7

Nondrug, Complementary, and Alternative Medicine Approaches to Pain Relief

Nurses have the knowledge and skill to use a variety of pain-relief strategies. Some techniques do require prescriptions, referrals, or highly technical procedures; while others are within the scope of nursing practice. The focus of this chapter will be on interventions that are safe, noninvasive, and require little, if any, technology.

Nondrug* interventions often are categorized as conventional medicine, complementary or alternative medicine, and integrative approaches.

Conventional Medicine

In the conventional medical system, nondrug pain relief methods are classified as physical or psychosocial (cognitive/behavioral) modalities [1].

Physical Modalities

Nurses instruct patients in the use of several conventional pain-relieving, self-management activities. These include:

- Positioning for comfort, alignment, and healing
- Good health practices, such as diet, exercise, fresh air, and ample sleep
- Graded activity, therapeutic exercises
- Breathing techniques
- Pacing activities while using proper body mechanics

---

*Nondrug is used synonymously with nonpharmacological in this text.

- Avoiding pain triggers
- Using medications, special dressings, and adaptive equipment

Psychosocial Modalities

Psychosocial modalities focus on altering the patient's thoughts, feelings, or behaviors. Nurses use many teaching and counseling strategies to help shape patients' understanding of their conditions, listen to their concerns, enhance coping, and lessen pain-related disability. Specific strategies include:

- Distract attention away from pain
  - Therapeutic humor
  - Conversations about what interests the patients
  - Read, listen to music, or pursue activities they enjoy
- Providing opportunity for private emotional disclosure
  - Private conversations that allow "safe" expression of feelings
  - Journal writing about feeling or bothersome situations
- Basic relaxation techniques

Mental health nurses or psychologists have a variety of techniques that are useful for patients with pain. Some psychological modalities requiring advanced skills that help control pain are:

- Biofeedback to regulate blood flow, heart rate, and muscle tension
- Advanced relaxation and imagery techniques
- Cognitive-behavioral therapy (e.g., learning to change thoughts, feelings, and behaviors)

 NURSE-TO-NURSE TIP

Teach activity pacing to patients to maximize functioning while reducing pain and the risk of injury. Break multistep activities into smaller parts, and consider ways to simplify or modify activities to reduce pain triggers. When starting the activity, and periodically thereafter, the patient notes the character and intensity of pain. When significant changes are noted (e.g., sudden shooting pain or increase in pain by 2 points on a 0–10 scale), the patient should stop or modify activity, allowing the pain to subside, then resume the activity or seek help. For example, a patient washing dishes notices after 5 minutes of standing, pain increases by 2 points and throbbing ensues. If repositioning (e.g., one foot on a step stool) is ineffective, the patient should sit for 15 minutes to allow pain to subside before resuming the activity. Help from another person may be sought for the most painful part (e.g., loading dishwasher or cleaning heavy pots) of the activity.

- Hypnoanalgesia and self-hypnosis
- Motivational interviewing
- Acceptance and commitment therapy

Behavioral Approaches

Some psychosocial approaches are directed toward behavioral changes. These may focus on the way persons living with pain fulfill their usual roles or relate with others. Some behavioral strategies helping people with pain include:

- Operant therapy (e.g., contingency management) that reinforces adaptive and extinguishes maladaptive pain behaviors
- Group therapy (e.g., psychotherapy, cognitive behavioral therapy)
- Work-hardening/functional restoration programs (develop strength, endurance and psychosocial capacity needed to return to work)

In addition to these pain-reducing psychosocial interventions, patients should receive mental health services to treat any comorbid psychological disorders (e.g., depression, post-traumatic stress disorder, etc.) that are identified.

Complementary and Alternative Medicine Approaches

Complementary therapies are generally used along with standard medical treatments, whereas alternative medicine approaches are used instead of conventional therapies. The National Institutes of Health defines complementary and alternative medicine (CAM) as "a broad domain of healing resources that encompasses health systems, modalities, and practices ... other than those intrinsic to the dominant system" [2, p. 1].

Given that broad definition, it is not surprising that Americans spend more money out of pocket on CAM therapies than they do on doctors or hospitalization [3]. Some of these techniques may cause adverse effects or interactions with medical therapies. Professionals need to ask patients about their use of these methods in a nonjudgmental manner. To help stimulate the research needed to establish CAM safety and efficacy, the National Institutes of Health established the National Center for Complementary and Alternative Medicine (NCCAM). They classify CAM (see Table 7–1) into five categories [4]:

- Alternative Medical Systems
- Mind-Body Medicine
- Biologically Based Therapy
- Manipulative and Body-Based Practices
- Energy-Based Medicine

Table 7–1 NCCAM Classification of CAM Interventions

CAM CLASSIFICATION	DESCRIPTION
Alternative Medical Systems	Whole medical systems with beliefs about health/disease (and treatments) that differ from conventional medicine
Homeopathy	Stimulates healing with highly dilute "like" substances
Traditional Chinese Medicine	Balance yin-and-yang energies (qi) with acupuncture, herbs, meditation, and massage
Ayurveda/Acupuncture	Balances mind, body, and spirit with herbs, yoga, and massage
Naturopathic Medicine	European-based approach to health using diet and lifestyle change plus herbs, massage, and joint manipulation
Mind-Body Medicine	Techniques that enhance the mind's capacity to affect bodily function and symptoms
Hypnosis	Suggestions made by therapist to facilitate change in health or comfort
Relaxation/Imagery Techniques	A variety of techniques designed to decrease and counteract the effects of stress
Cognitive-Behavioral Therapy	Therapeutic approach to change thoughts and behaviors believed to negatively affect health and worsen symptoms
Creative Outlets	Music, art, and dance used to promote health and symptom control
Biologic-Based Therapies	Use of substances found in nature
Diets	Use of certain diets (e.g., vegan, probiotic, macrobiotic, etc.) to affect health
Herbal Supplements	Plant products believed to have medicinal values
Vitamin	Use of vitamins/minerals (often in high doses) to promote health or prevent/treat disease

Table 7–1 NCCAM Classification of CAM Interventions—cont'd

CAM CLASSIFICATION	DESCRIPTION
Manipulation/Body-Based Therapy	Based on manipulation or movement of body parts
Chiropractic	Realignment of subluxated areas of the spine to promote health and treat symptoms
Massage Therapy	Pressing, rubbing, moving tissue to improve circulation, health, and comfort
Osteopathic Medicine	Form of manipulation performed by doctor of osteopathic medicine, used in conjunction with physical therapy
Energy Therapies	Therapeutic use of biofield or electromagnetic energy
Reiki	Channeling of healing energy through a Reiki practitioner
Magnetic Therapy	Use of magnets or electromagnetic fields for health

NCCAM—National Center for Complementary and Alternative Medicine; CAM—Complementary and Alternative Medicine. Adapted from NCCAM Web site, http://nccam.nih.gov/health/whatiscam/overview.htm

Many nurses have embraced selected CAM therapies, because they are aligned with valued concepts of holism and humanism. Nurses should become knowledgeable about CAM therapies because of their prevalent use (by 35% to 60% of patients), their potential to cut pain or anxiety, while improving coping, sleep, and quality of life. Nurses also should understand CAM therapy because their use may be counterproductive or contraindicated in combination with particular medicines or diagnoses. Occasionally, CAM providers may further distance patients from mainstream medicine by reinforcing inaccurate notions about potential harm and ineffectiveness of conventional

GENERAL: CAM

Many people turn to CAM to give them a greater sense of control so they no longer feel dependent on a doctor, a pill, or a procedure. Pain is the most common reason why people use CAM approaches [5], which usually are used in conjunction with medical treatments. Close to 40% of patients however, seek CAM therapies because of
Continued

a failure to benefit from conventional medicine or a lack of access to medicine. Patients also may choose CAM therapy if they receive more attentive, personalized, unhurried care than what is provided by their doctor.

therapies; while touting the safety of their therapy and failing to disclose that injury, illness, and even deaths have resulted from CAM treatments [5].

Alternative Medical Systems

Many alternative medical systems have a long history and a track record of success with impressive case reports. Ancient systems, such as traditional Chinese medicine or Ayurvedic medicine from India have been refining their treatments for centuries. The view of health as a balance is an important theme in these and more contemporary "alternative" systems. Many alternative systems use herbal treatments, defending their safety compared with modern drugs. However, more than 20% of the Ayurvedic "natural" products tested contained toxic levels of lead, mercury, or arsenic [6]. Similarly, nearly one-third of Chinese herbal products tested contained prescription drugs or toxic metal contamination [7].

Naturopathy and homeopathy are alternative medical systems developed in the 18th and 19th centuries based on a premise of providing the body what it needs for self-healing. Naturopathy, originally with roots in conventional medicine, can include a variety of treatments directed at the assumed cause (not symptom), such as the need for specialized diets, botanicals, acupuncture, physical medicine, and psychological counseling.

In contrast, homeopathy was born out of an opposition to the dangers of traditional medicine. The underlying homeopathic belief maintains that "like heals like." Therefore pain-producing substances are needed to heal pain. Naturally irritating substances, such as capsaicin or Arnica montana are used for pain. What is considered by mainstream medicine to be the high-strength (1%) capsaicin (derived from jalapeño peppers) would be deemed low potency from the homeopathic perspective. By homeopathic principles, further diluting and shaking 1 part capsaicin in 99 parts water adds potency. For the best effect, a standard homeopathic preparation would undergo 30 serial dilutions. Conventional medicine routinely dismisses these therapies as deriving their benefit from nothing more than a placebo effect, despite at least one placebo-controlled trial supporting the superiority of some homeopathic remedies [8].

A recent systematic research review focused on the use of CAM for neuropathic pain. Only 20 trials and systematic reviews qualified for this rigorous review. Mixed results for neuropathic pain were reported for acupuncture and herbal therapy. Spiritual healing and Saint John's wort did not have pain-relieving effects. However, capsaicin and acetyl-L-carnitine (levacecarnine), geranium oil, magnets, and imagery showed evidence of relieving neuropathic pain [9].

Mind-Body Interventions

Mind-body approaches focus on the interactions between the mind (i.e., thoughts, feelings, and attitudes), behavior, and physical health. They emphasize mastering self-regulation to mobilize innate healing powers through self-knowledge and self-care. Common methods of accessing these healing powers include:

- Relaxation, meditation, or prayer quiets the mind and body to allow healing to take place
- Guided imagery uses mentally created images to produce physiological change
- Biofeedback teaches control of bodily functions one is normally unaware of
- Cognitive-behavioral therapy promotes coping skill mastery and a self-discovery process

Mind-body medicine has an impressive body of research supporting its use, with a 1996 National Institute of Health Technology Assessment Panel urging health professionals to use these therapies more for patients with chronic pain. Benefits include a reduction in health-care visits, improved coping, and reductions in pain, disability, and depression [10–12], using techniques within the scope of nursing practice [13].

Biological-Based Therapies

Biological-based therapies use natural substances to promote comfort and health. Many patients use these therapies, often without considering them to be a treatment. Some may interact with conventional medical therapies in a potentially harmful way. Examples include:

- Herbs, such as Saint John's wort, alter blood levels and metabolism of drugs (e.g., methadone)
- Food supplements, such as glucosamine, devil's claw, and S-adenosylmethionine (SAM-e)

- These supplements are the best studied and likely provide some benefit [14]
  - SAM-e may interact with serotonergic drugs
- Supplemental vitamins B, C, D, and E have relieved specific types of pain
- A diet rich in omega-3 fatty acids *and* lower in omega-6 fats to reduce inflammatory pain

Other herbal or nutritional supplements are used for pain, but have less evidence of benefit including:

- Echinacea: for pain associated with inflammation or advanced states of disease
- Kava: for pain and insomnia; may damage the liver
- Meadowsweet: for abdominal pain; produces salicylic acid (aspirin precursor)
- Willow bark: for pain, inflammation and infections; salicylic acid interacts with aspirin
- Pau d'arco: for pain, infection and other diseases; provides blood-thinning effect
- Turmeric: for pain associated with inflammation; may have antineoplastic properties

Manipulative and Body-Based Practices

Manipulative and body-based practices are believed to relieve pain on the basis that adjustment or alignment of one body part helps promote or restore health. Massage therapy, chiropractic care, reflexology, and osteopathic medicine are the most common forms of this type of approach. Lesser known methods include:

- Rolfing: deep-tissue body work (myofascial release) and movement education
- Bowen technique: gentle intermittent movement of specific muscles and tissues
- Trager work: relaxation and gentle movement
- Alexander and Feldenkrais methods: gentle, poised, tailored mindful movements
- Craniosacral massage: light touch along the axial plane, skull to sacrum

Massage therapy and chiropractic care are the most popular methods and have compelling evidence of pain relief benefits. Massage is the more effective of the two and is useful for more pain types [15]. Patients who are very ill or frail and those with osteoporosis are at greatest risk of being injured with these methods, which are otherwise considered quite safe [16].

Energy Medicine

Two types of energy may be targeted for the transfer of energy by human or mechanical means:

- Veritable energy is objectively measurable (sound, light, magnets)
- Putative energy has no accepted objective form of measurement (biofield, Ch'i)

From an energy perspective, pain can represent a deficiency, excess, or impeded flow of energy. Adjustment can be accomplished by modifying or redirecting energy fields that surround and penetrate the body. Some techniques require physical contact or penetration of the body (i.e., acupuncture, some forms of Reiki). Other adjustments manipulate energy fields (i.e., aura or chakras) inches above the body's surface. Distance healing can be done through some forms (i.e., Reiki, healing intent, prayer, etc.) of energy medicine.

Some energy medicine modalities are very prescriptive (specific time exposed to light using precise frequencies), whereas others (Qi gong, therapeutic touch) involve a dynamic evaluation and adjustment of subjectively perceived energy fields. Specific modalities listed by NCCAM under the umbrella of energy medicine that are used for pain include:

- Intercessory prayer: praying on behalf of another
- Reiki: universal energy source directed by healer's hands
- Qi gong: breathing and movement exercises that circulate *qi* (Ch'i) through meridians
- Healing touch: practitioner's gentle use of hands to repattern patients' energy field
- Acupuncture: inserting and manipulating fine needles to direct *qi* through meridians
- Magnets: use of pulsed electromagnetic fields or static, topically positioned magnets
- Sound (music) therapy: specific sound frequencies and rhythms used for health

COACH CONSULT

What is Reiki? *Rei* and *Ki* are Japanese characters signifying "universal" and "life energy." Illness and its symptoms are seen as manifestations of low energy. Different forms of Reiki resemble "laying on of hands," therapeutic touch, and distance healing techniques. The Reiki practitioner becomes attuned to universal energy sources and promotes the flow of energy needed for healing and symptom reduction. Treatments can last an hour, as the universal life energy is allowed to do its work.

- Light therapy: use of high-intensity lights or low-level lasers

Within these methods, certain related techniques may be used for pain:

- Pain-drain form of healing touch removes and replaces pain with comforting energy [17]
- Moxibustion: practitioner burns dried herbs (moxa) and either uses them to warm the acupuncture sites (with or without needles in place)

Evidence of Safety and Efficacy of CAM Therapies

Despite the widespread popular use of CAM therapies for pain control, research that meets the highest standards of quality is limited. Many CAM therapies cannot achieve the level of evidence deemed necessary by mainstream medicine to support their safe, effective use because of difficulties performing randomized, double-blind, placebo-controlled trials. Challenges abound for investigators developing models of blinding or placebo controls, especially for alternative medical systems and therapies that use putative energy sources.

Given limited evidence of the safety and efficacy for many specific CAM techniques, their routine use cannot be recommended as a substitute for conventional medicine. This is especially true for patients with life-limiting diseases, such as cancer, who can easily develop serious complications. Knowledge of what the specific treatments entail and related risks will help the nurse counsel patients about their use. As with pharmacological therapy, evaluate patient response during and just after treatments, especially the initial one. After a few sessions, most patients will be able to evaluate the relative costs and benefits of a particular therapy and decide whether or not to continue.

Integrative Approaches to Pain Relief

Integrative medicine "takes into account the whole person (mind, body, and spirit)... and makes use of all appropriate therapies, both conventional and alternative" [18, p. 7] to optimize health. That definition, combined with the long-accepted definition of health as: "a state of complete physical, mental and social well-being" [19, p. 1], suggests that comprehensive care attends to the mind, body, spirit, and social interactions. Patients benefit by combining a variety of techniques, especially when pain is severe or persistent. Ideally, these combinations simultaneously target biopsychosocial and spiritual needs. Integrated techniques using both multimodal pharmacological and nondrug techniques have demonstrated their efficacy and cost-effectiveness for many years [11, 20–22].

Active Versus Passive Techniques

Passive treatments, such as healing touch, acupuncture, and chiropractic manipulation require the patient to be a submissive recipient of treatment. Using only passive forms of therapy may reinforce feelings of powerlessness and put the onus of responsibility for pain control on the professional. Active self-management techniques must be included in the treatment plan of a patient who is able to do things on his or her own behalf [23]. Active techniques, in the form of mastered self-initiated skills (e.g., pacing activities, self-massage, or self-hypnosis) can be available where and when the patient needs to control the pain. The use of self-initiated techniques alone may not be sufficient to control the pain. Combined with professional interventions however, they can have a synergistic rather than a mere additive effect [24].

Providing pain relief in a comprehensive, integrative manner requires the nurse to know the patient's pain from the perspective of the mind, body, spirit, and social interactions. The assessment chapter (Chapter 4) of this book delineates a structure for the nurse.

Selected Nondrug Techniques

Table 7–2 lists interventions that target the mind, body, spirit, and social domains. Remember that a given intervention may target multiple domains simultaneously. When pain is severe or chronic, a combination of interventions is needed.

Table 7–2 Noninvasive Nondrug Treatment Options by Target

DOMAIN OF PAIN	TREATMENT APPROACH
Body	Reducing pain triggers Massage, self-massage Applying heat or ice TENS Positioning, use of brace/orthotics Acupressure Diet, nutritional supplements Exercise: stretching, strengthening, endurance Pacing activities, yoga Sleep hygiene Cutaneous stimulation
Mind	Relaxation, imagery, mindfulness Self-hypnosis

Continued

Table 7–2 **Noninvasive Nondrug Treatment Options by Target—cont'd**

DOMAIN OF PAIN	TREATMENT APPROACH
Mind (cont'd)	Pain diary, journal writing Distracting attention Repattern thinking Attitude adjustment Reduce fear, anxiety, stress Reduce sadness, helplessness Learn more about own pain/relief
Spirit	Prayer, meditation Self-reflection, narratives (e.g., life/pain) Meaningful rituals Energy work (e.g., TT*, Reiki)
Social Interactions	Function at highest level possible Improved communication Optimize family relations Problem-solving Volunteering Support groups

*TT—Therapeutic Touch

Selected Nondrug Interventions Directed at the Body

Cutaneous Stimulation

In addition to thermotherapy and massage (detailed below); vibration, tapping, electrical stimulation, and applying pressure are commonly used methods of stimulation. High-frequency vibration is helpful and can be applied using handheld devices or be integrated into a chair or mattress. Stimulation can be applied at different places and still be effective [25], including:

- Directly on or near the pain
- Proximal to the pain—between the pain and brain
- Distal to the pain—past the pain along the nerve path (dermatome)
- At acupuncture/acupressure points
- Contralateral to the pain—exact location, opposite side of the body

Cutaneous stimulation may aggravate pain in some people, especially those with migraine headaches or very sensitive skin, such as allodynia or a burn. Avoid cutaneous stimulation at areas of infection, damaged skin, or over thrombophlebitis. Take care to prevent injury for those with neurological deficits in the area being stimulated and in patients who bruise easily. Indirect (e.g., contralateral or proximal) stimulation can be useful when the painful area is hypersensitive, inaccessible by a cast or bandages, or missing (phantom pain). Transcutaneous electrical nerve stimulation (TENS) is typically applied directly over or around areas of pain; but also can be applied to other locations, except the head* and chest, or over implanted devices.

Massage

Massage can aid physical and mental relaxation, cut muscle tension and spasms, and improve circulation and lymphatic flow. The most common forms of massage are:

- Petrissage—squeezing, rolling, and kneading muscles
- Effleurage—smooth gliding strokes
- Trigger-point release—concentrated pressure to painful, knotted muscles

Typically, an unscented hypoallergenic cream is used to reduce friction. Essential oils with comforting aromas or medicated liniments may provide additional localized relief of joint or muscle pain. Massage should be avoided in areas where there is inflammation, infection, tissue damage, and nerve or bone anomalies. It is generally contraindicated in areas of altered skin integrity (including fresh surgical incisions), over implanted devices, or near blood clots and tumors. Potentially violent patients or those who exhibit inappropriate sexual behaviors are not suitable candidates. Patients with hyperalgesia or allodynia may experience an increase in pain during the procedure, so it is important to discuss the patient's response. Attending to modesty needs, ambient temperature, lighting, and noise level is important, as these influence the patient's response. Massage has a growing body of literature supporting its utility to provide relief for a variety of painful conditions [26–28].

Application of Heat or Cold

Thermotherapy (therapeutic use of hot or cold) can be used at the site of pain or at proximal, distal, contralateral, or acupressure points. It may work by improving circulation and relaxing muscles. In contrast, cold decreases swelling, constricts blood vessels, and slows or blocks the transmission of pain impulses. With either type of application, there is a need to protect patients from thermal injury, especially those who are frail or have neurological deficits.

---

*TENS can be used on the forehead. Transcranial electrical stimulation devices use different current patterns than those used in other areas of the body.

Heat improves circulation and relaxes muscle; however it also can enhance swelling, metabolism, and inflammation. Heat applications also can have a cooling effect on the core temperature as surface vasodilation increases heat loss. The application of cold constricts blood vessels, which prevents swelling and suppresses inflammation, but it may cause shivering, muscle tension, or spasms. Combined with the vasoconstriction effect, core body temperature may rise with the application of cold packs or ice. In head-to-head trials for the treatment of pain, cold packs beat heat for arthritis pain and functioning [31], while heat was superior to either cold or nonopioid medications for acute (but not chronic) low back pain [32, 33].

Heat or cold can be applied in a variety of ways, including immersion of part or all of the body in water, heating or cooling blankets, gel packs, or wraps. Generally, the thermal source needs to remain in place for at least 10 minutes, with most applications achieving benefit in 20 to 30 minutes. Patients who have more subcutaneous fat may need longer applications. Mechanical devices are available, such as Cryo Cuff products by Aircast for applying cold; and ultrasound, diathermy, or paraffin treatments to deliver heat. These devices provide focused thermotherapy with better tissue-penetrating capacity than traditional methods of applying hot or cold packs.

Specific Precautions When Using Superficial Heat

Superficial heat modalities are contraindicated in the following situations:

- Hydrotherapy is contraindicated with surgical or open wounds, whether clean or infected
- Warm-water immersion elevates core body temperature, and is avoided in patients who have multiple sclerosis, adrenal insufficiency, lupus, or who are pregnant
- Radiant heat should not be used in patients with the following conditions:
  - Photosensitivity
  - Acute inflammation or hemorrhage
  - Bleeding disorder
  - Decreased sensation

- Do not use heat on ischemic part, because it increases metabolism and worsens ischemia
- Cleanse skin to remove applied oils or gels that can increase the risk of burns
- Avoid electric heating pads/blankets because of associated electrocution and fire risk

Specific Precautions When Using Superficial Cold

Avoid using superficial cold use in patients with the following conditions:

- Hypertension (due to secondary vasoconstriction)
- Raynaud's disease
- Rheumatoid arthritis
- Local limb ischemia
- History of vascular impairment, such as frostbite or arteriosclerosis
- Cold allergy (cold urticaria)
- Paroxysmal cold hemoglobinuria
- Cryoglobulinemia or any disease that produces a marked cold-pressor response

Cold packs applied to the abdomen also can cause increased gastrointestinal motility and gastric acid secretion; therefore, this treatment is contraindicated in those with known peptic ulcer disease. The application of hot packs to the abdomen produces the opposite effect, thus it may be beneficial when slowed motility and fewer secretions are desired, unless otherwise contraindicated.

Positioning for Optimal Comfort and Function

Immobilizing or restricting the movement of a painful body part promotes comfort and healing. Splints or supportive devices should hold joints in the position of optimal function and should be removed regularly to provide skin care and range-of-motion exercises. Prolonged immobilization can result in skin breakdown, joint contracture, muscle atrophy, bone demineralization, and cardiovascular problems. Patients should be encouraged to participate in self-care activities while remaining as active and strong as possible.

From the conventional medicine perspective, specific positions (e.g., semi-Fowler's, Sims', side-lying, etc.) may be indicated to promote comfort and well-being for patients with certain medical conditions. Lying on the right side may be most comfortable with gastrointestinal disorders; lying on the left side is best during pregnancy. Many CAM approaches—such as chiropractic care, Rolfing, Feldenkrais, Trager, and yoga—are based on the premise that repositioning, realignment, or learning proper posture and movements can relieve pain.

NURSE-TO-NURSE TIP

Some pain triggers, such as procedural pain, can be prevented by preemptive analgesia. Other pain triggers may be more subtle or insidious. Factors, such as bright fluorescent lighting, eating foods high in sugars, omega-6 fatty acids, salts, or additives such as aspartame can worsen pain for some patients. Too much or too little exercise can put the patient at risk for injury or for developing painful muscle spasms. Given that too much or too little sleep can trigger headaches or increase next-day pain, sleep hygiene can be added to the list of nursing interventions that lower pain.

Selected Nondrug Interventions Directed at the Mind

The goals of nursing the mind include promoting comfort, alleviating suffering, reducing physiological and mental triggers/amplifiers of pain, and optimizing functioning. See Table 7–2 for a list of techniques that help patients to accomplish these goals.

Distraction

Distraction draws the person's attention away from his or her pain, reducing its acuity. There are different forms of distraction, but the best distraction is interactive, situation-specific based on the individual's interests, preferences, energy level, and ability-to-focus attention. Common forms of distraction may be considered based on the primary sense being stimulated, such as:

- Visual distraction—reading, viewing art/photography, and watching TV or a movie
- Auditory distraction—listening to music, talk-radio, books on tape
- Olfactory distraction—aroma therapy
- Tactile distraction—caring touch, pet therapy

Using multiple forms of distraction simultaneously adds value to the activity (e.g., listening to music while tapping to the music, singing along, or playing along on a musical instrument). Engaging multiple senses simultaneously can help, as can engaging the mind in other than sensory ways. Watching a favorite TV show or favorite sports team, or listening to one's favorite song has much better distraction value than watching or listening to something with less personal interest. Activities that pose intellectual, social, or motor-skill challenges can have a high distraction value (e.g., puzzles, interactive games, or hobbies).

Simple distraction techniques, such as counting, are quite beneficial during brief episodes of procedural pain. With more severe or persistent pain, multisensory, biopsychosocial forms are more effective. At times, patients may distract their attention from pain so effectively that they overexert and injure themselves unknowingly. Guide patients to pay attention to signals indicating a worsening of pain and respect for their activity-restriction limits.

Relaxation Techniques

Stress is known to boost pain by increasing muscle tension, activating the sympathetic nervous system, and putting the patient at risk for stress-related pain (tension headaches). Eliciting the relaxation response decreases and counteracts the harmful effects of stress. Common relaxation techniques include progressive relaxation, breath-focused relaxation, and meditation (see Table 7–3). The nurse can help elicit the relaxation response by verbal coaching, teaching simple self-directed meditation, or providing audio or audiovisual recordings. Boxes 7–1 to 7–3 provide sample scripts nurses can use to coach relaxation. In general, basic relaxation techniques do not yield remarkable pain-relief although they reduce the amplification of pain created by physical or mental stress. Once the patient has mastered the basic skills, advanced techniques, such as guided imagery or self-hypnosis can be used to change the pain intensity, distribution, or character of pain [34].

Table 7–3 Common Types of Relaxation Techniques

RELAXATION TECHNIQUE NAME	DESCRIPTION
Diaphragmatic Breathing	Take in slow, deep breaths through the nose. Pause, and then breathe out through the mouth. Exhalation takes twice as long as inhalation to expel as much air as possible. Do five breath sets. Learn to isolate the diaphragm by placing one hand on the abdomen—and the other on the chest. Practice "belly breathing" until only the hand on abdomen moves.
Progressive Muscle Relaxation	Actively tense and relax various muscle groups to discriminate feelings of tension from those of relaxation. After tensing and relaxing all major muscle groups from head to toe, (or toe to head) focus on making muscle groups increasingly relaxed. Eventually, focusing only on relaxation.

Continued

Nondrug, Complementary, and Alternative Medicine Approaches to Pain Relief **167**

Table 7–3 Common Types of Relaxation Techniques—cont'd

RELAXATION TECHNIQUE NAME	DESCRIPTION
Autogenic (Modified Progressive) Relaxation	Similar to progressive muscle relaxation, without actively tensing muscle groups. Instead focus on creating a desired state (warm, heavy, relaxed muscles) in successive muscle groups. Then focus on areas where tension remains.
Mindful Meditation	A body-scan technique similar to autogenic relaxation. Focus on all sensations felt in each body part with a nonjudgmental, accepting attitude. For example: areas of soreness, burning, or throbbing are mentally identified and accepted "as is" while letting go of any related sadness or anger (see Table 7–4 on page 172) and learning to better understand and control the sensation.
Transcendental Meditation (TM) Relaxation Response (RR)	Repeat a mantra (in TM) or alternative mental focus (in RR), such as a word, phrase, sound, or prayer. Let go of other thoughts that distract from that focus (passive attitude). This repetition continues for at least 20 min.
Pleasant Imagery	After a body-scan technique similar to autogenic (above), generate mental images of a place deemed comfortable, safe, or special. Images include pleasant sights, sounds, and smells associated with that desirable real or imaginary place.
Guided Imagery	Working with a therapist, patient forms an image representing the pain or its cause. Patient then uses his or her imagination to attack the cause or improve comfort. This is done by using images that represent normal processes such as releasing endorphins or mobilizing immune cells.
Hypnosis	A state of deep relaxation and altered consciousness that produces a heightened receptiveness to suggestion. Typical steps include deep relaxation, attention fixation, suggestion of desired change (immediate and delayed), and restoration of fully conscious, aware state.

Box 7–1 Breath-Focused Relaxation*

Beginning

Take a deep abdominal breath in through your nose ... hold it a moment ... now breathe out completely through pursed lips ... then just allow your breath to come naturally to you.

As you breathe in ... invite its nourishing warmth into all parts of your body ... or, you may direct your breath to parts of your body that need comforting.

As you breathe out, let the tension go ... into the room where it disappears.

Allow any tension you are aware of to flow out with each out breath ...

Pause after each out-breath until the next in-breath is ready to begin ...

Middle

As you breathe in ... say to yourself, "in, 2, 3" As you breathe out ... say to yourself, "out, 2, 3."

Simply focus on your breath ... on the in-breath ... on the out-breath ... or on both ... *[long pause]* ... If you become distracted by your thoughts, simply go back to your focus *[long pause]*. If you have become distracted, gently guide your awareness back to your focus *[pause]*.

End

Gently bring your awareness back ... being more aware of your surroundings knowing that you can return to this relaxed state whenever you choose. When ready, open your eyes, feeling relaxed and refreshed.

*Reproduced with permission of Margaret Caudill-Slosberg, MD, MPH, author of *Managing Pain Before It Manages You, Third Edition*, Guilford Press, 2009.

Box 7–2 Brief Autogenic Body-Scan Relaxation*

Beginning: Use the beginning from breath-focused relaxation technique. (See Box 7–1)

Middle

Direct the comfort of your in-breath to the top of your head, your forehead, around your eyes ... and breathe out the tension.

Notice any area of tension in your jaw, cheeks, lips, and tongue. Let them soften and relax as you breathe out the tension...

Let your shoulders drop slightly as you allow warm, soft, heavy relaxed feelings to be felt in your head, face, neck, and shoulders.

Let the tension go from your right arm ... and your left arm ... letting the tension go from your upper arms, elbows, forearms, wrists, hands, and fingers ... just let the tension go.

Continued

Nondrug, Complementary, and Alternative Medicine Approaches to Pain Relief **169**

Box 7–2 Brief Autogenic Body-Scan Relaxation*—cont'd

Direct the comfort of your in-breath to any areas of tension in your torso... chest, abdomen, pelvis, and back. Let the comfort of your in-breath surround the area of tension, soften it ... and breathe out the tension.

Let the tension go from your right leg .... And your left leg ... including the buttocks, hips, thighs, calves, ankles, feet, and toes ... just let the tension go.

Now take a moment to direct the comfort of your in-breath to any area where tension remains. Let the comfort of your in-breath surround the area of tension, soften it ... and breathe out the tension. Each time you breathe out feel yourself going deeper into a state of inner peace and calm.

End: Use the ending from breath-focused relaxation technique. (See Box 7–1)

*Reproduced with permission of Margaret Caudill-Slosberg, MD, MPH, author of *Managing Pain Before It Manages You, Third Edition*, Guilford Press, 2009.

Box 7–3 Pleasant Imagery-assisted Relaxation*

Beginning: Start with the beginning of breath-focused–relaxation technique and a brief body scan. (See Boxes 7–1 and 7–2)

Middle

Now imagine yourself in a beautiful meadow ... sun shining overhead ... not too hot ... not too cool ... a gentle breeze blows across your body.

In the distance you can hear birds singing ... and the wind in the nearby trees ... the fragrance of flowers fills the air as you move effortlessly along the path ...

This path takes you to a special place ... a place that you equate with peace ... quiet ... and tranquility ... a safe haven ... it can be a favorite place where you live ... a place and time that was relaxing, safe, or special ... or a place that you would like to go to in the future...

It can be a fantasy place, created entirely by the powers of your imagination... Take this time to create a safe, special place for yourself...

Imagine the sights you would see ... the colors, textures, details ... the sounds you would hear ... the fragrances you might smell ... the gentle coolness of a breeze, or warmth of the sun on your skin as you imagine settling into a comfortable position ...

Box 7–3 **Pleasant Imagery-assisted Relaxation*—cont'd**

Now, while in this place of peace and tranquility, turn the focus of your attention on your breath, a word or phrase ... on the in-breath ... on the out-breath ... or on both.... *(long pause)* ...If you become distracted by your thoughts, simply go back to your focus *(long pause)*. If you have become distracted, gently guide your awareness back to your focus *(pause)*.

End: Use the ending from the breath-focused relaxation technique. (See Box 7–1)

*Reproduced with permission of Margaret Caudill-Slosberg, MD, MPH, author of *Managing Pain Before It Manages You, Third Edition,* Guilford Press, 2009.

Table 7–4 **Cost-Benefit Analysis: Holding Onto Anger**

After the patient understands that he or she feels anger, brainstorm the costs and benefits:

COST OF BEING ANGRY	BENEFIT OF BEING ANGRY
Tension headaches Heart races Blood pressure increases Risk of stroke/heart attack Muscle spasm Increases back pain Family avoids talking Family avoids doing things together Friends do not call	I am left alone. I have energy to get up and get things done. I want the person to realize they hurt me. I want the person who hurt me to pay for what he or she did.

After brainstorming, ask patient if anger is costing more that it is benefiting.
Consider ways to let go of anger or forgive the person(s) whom is the source of anger to lower the cost of being angry.
Consider using the energy from anger in a single goal-directed way to maximize the potential benefit. After the expression of anger to the appropriate person, let the anger go. Continuing to hold onto and express anger increases the cost and diminishes the possibility of benefit.

Relaxation techniques generally are safe, although precautions are required for some patients. For example, those who have been victimized or who have mental health disorders may become disturbed by intrusive thoughts or images. For these patients it is recommended that trained mental health professionals perform these procedures. These techniques need to be used cautiously in patients with unstable cardiovascular or respiratory status. Other precautious include the need to avoid images of warmth in areas of the body that are actively bleeding. It is best, when using pleasant imagery, to allow patients to create the images from their own experiences rather than the professional's idea of a relaxing image. For example, while a beach scene may be relaxing to the nurse, a patient may associate a beach with a traumatic event.

Facilitating Coping

Using therapeutic communication, nurses can help patients who are anxious, sad, grieving, overly pessimistic, or helpless. Therapeutic communication emphasizes active listening, encouragement, problem-solving, and empathy. To promote active self-care, nurses often facilitate coping by:

- Exploring and allowing the expression of feelings
- Goal setting and problem-solving
- Facilitating communication with others (including rehearsal of difficult conversations)
- Providing patient education and counseling
- Facilitating access to needed resources

For patients with severe emotional distress, counseling from trained professionals is indicated.

Patient education about pain and its treatment helps alleviate pain, either through a reduction of anxiety or enhanced adherence with the treatment plan. Nurses also can help by recognizing and challenging thought patterns known to worsen pain, disability, and despair. Particularly problematic are: strong self-doubts, unrealistic expectations, helplessness, rumination, or catastrophic-thinking patterns [35, 36].

Positive self-statements or affirmations, such as "I can handle this...," "I'm doing the best I can...," and "I am becoming stronger" can help the patient change unhelpful attitudes. When a patient is immobilized by strong emotions, such as anger, a cost-benefit analysis may help him or her cope better (see Box 7–1).

Selected Nondrug Interventions Directed at the Spirit

The goal of spiritual interventions include: the reduction of spiritual distress and existential suffering. Ultimately, this can dampen pain amplifiers

---

🐦 NURSE-TO-NURSE TIP

Nurses can help patients interfere with the harmful effects of errant thinking through the use of a "thought-stopping" procedure. Whenever the patient becomes overly pessimistic, teach him or her to stop those thoughts and take a deep diaphragmatic breath. Help the patient recognize thoughts that are not true and are not helpful. Help the patient restate the current situation with realistic, adaptive, and confidence-building thoughts. When the thought is successfully challenged, the patient should feel immediate relief of emotional distress [37, 38].

NURSE-TO-NURSE TIP

Jumping to conclusions can increase pain and distress: Mrs. Tandy was upset by the thought "I'll never dance again," a statement she was convinced was true. Exploring the underlying assumptions linked to that statement revealed that her connection to the dance club was her only means of socializing. Beneath this thought lay the immobilizing fear that her social life would be ruined and she would be left alone. Once she was encouraged to explore other ways of socializing, she could take steps to think, feel, and do better [39].

to diminish its perception, while optimizing functioning and quality of life. The spiritual dimension encompasses a person's innermost concerns and values, including the ascribed purpose, meaning, and driving force of life. It may or may not be religious in nature. It may include rituals that help the individual feel part of a community, or a bond with something larger than themselves (i.e., God, nature, or the universe). Interventions directed at the spiritual domain flow from the spiritual assessment. The nurse may ask questions, such as:

- Is religion or spirituality a source of strength or comfort to you during difficult times?
- What aspects of your religion or spirituality do you find most helpful?
- Do your religious or spiritual beliefs affect the kind of care you would like to receive?

The care plan should reflect the patient's spiritual needs, resources, and spiritual care preferences.

Prayer

For patients expressing their spirituality in a religious context, offering prayer or inspirational readings may help. For some patients, viewing meaningful religious symbols has been found to lower pain perception [40]. Patients may want to pray in private, pray with others, or be prayed for (intercessory prayer). Alternatively, they may want access to meaningful rituals (e.g., rosary beads, Communion, sunrise meditation, etc.). Although clinical pastoral education trains chaplains to facilitate prayer and spiritual care to patients from a variety of religious backgrounds [41], patients may feel best served by a particular spiritual-care provider. Facilitating access to that provider is an important nursing role.

Healing Touch

Many religious traditions include rituals that combine prayer with healing touch. Some holistic traditions view humans as irreducible energy fields that interact with universal sources of energy. A spiritual approach to pain control may take the form of simple touch or manipulation of energy patterns, whether or not it is part of a religious ritual. Therapeutic touch is one example of a nonreligious method nurses use to comfort by changing a patient's energy flow [42–46]. The patient may lie down or sit in a chair while the nurse/healer progresses through the following steps:

- Healer centers, and quiets self
- Healer focuses on the patient and the intent to help
- Healer assesses a patient's body by moving hands in a sweeping motion (light touch or noncontact) from head to feet
- Healer notices differences (accumulated, depleted, or asymmetric) in the energy field
- Healer performs hand movements to unruffle, unblock, or change the energy pattern
- Healer ensures smooth, symmetric energy flow with final sweeps

Personal Narratives

Personal narratives inform nurses about the patients' perception of their suffering, their hopes, and how illness has affected them. Written narratives, especially those high in emotional disclosure, produce significant reductions in pain [48]. Narratives help patients make sense of their lives and current situations; provide insights into their needs; and show how health decisions may affect their physical, mental, and spiritual well-being [49]. Composing a narrative may help by permitting the patient to make sense of the pain and understand how it relates to the meaning or purpose in his or her life. The narrative may focus on a turning point or on a specific event or feeling. When patients share their insights, they often experience a strong sense of relief. Caution is advised in using this technique with patients having post-traumatic stress disorder, who may need skilled counseling to deal with the flood of emotions triggered by their disclosure.

EVIDENCE FOR PRACTICE

Many techniques attempt to heal through the direction of energy. A randomized controlled trial (RCT) comparing two such healers from different traditions showed that one healer achieved significant, lasting pain reduction and functional improvement. However, the research could not determine whether the benefits were related to the specific technique or the skill of the healer [47].

Selected Nondrug Interventions Directed at Social Interactions

The goals of interventions targeting social interactions include restoring the person's place within family, community, and social network to the greatest extent possible, while fostering independence. This will reduce a major source of suffering that can amplify pain and despair.

Given the demoralizing and debilitating effects of severe or chronic pain, patients often withdraw socially and eventually lose the connections and support of family and friends. Sometimes the person with pain yearns for human contact, but even simple touch can send shock waves of pain through his or her body. Many patients need to find ways to repair damaged relationships, develop new associations, and resume active roles. At home, financial and workload burdens create tensions that demand honest, open, assertive communication. As a patient advocate, the nurse can contribute by helping patients improve communication with family members. In some cases, a family counselor or mediator is needed to solve deeply rooted problems. If pain interferes with the ability to work, an additional layer of problems and interpersonal tensions is created. Sadly, return to work and functional restoration programs often fall short of a person's goals after a pain-producing injury [50].

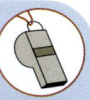

COACH CONSULT

Spiritual distress manifests itself in different ways, especially at the end of life. Pain and suffering are a sign of spiritual distress, as is a sense of emptiness and questioning one's own belief system. To reduce spiritual distress nurses can help patients feel at peace by allowing them to tell their story and express uncertainty; explore the meaning of illness; help them gain a sense of control; and offer assistance with prayer or meaningful rituals.

Caring and Therapeutic Presence

For those with pain, caring presence, attentive listening, and facilitating the process of acceptance can help. In one of the first research studies of nondrug pain relief measures, nursing interaction helped patients in pain feel better [51]. The presence of another person had an affect on the perception of pain; a caring presence was best able to provide relief [51]. The combination of caring presence and active listening is known to alleviate suffering. When there is no available drug or surgery to cure a patient's pain, human compassion and unconditional regard for the person's worth can make a difference.

The beneficial placebo effect is believed to be the result of effective therapeutic relationships, and has been dubbed the "healer effect" by some [52]. Its comforting and healing power may be active in all therapies, especially when the provider is friendly, warm, concerned, sympathetic, empathetic, prestigious, thorough, and competent [52, 53]. As a nurse, consider the potential benefits of spending a few minutes during each patient encounter developing trust and confidence. Rapport, confidence in the diagnostic label, and enthusiasm for the treatment are believed to enhance clinical outcomes [54].

Support Groups

Support groups can provide people with pain an opportunity to come together, share their experiences, and learn in setting where they have some power or control. Chronic pain patients attending either "educational" or "professionally led" support groups have been shown to do better in the area of sick-role behaviors than those without support groups [55]. Support group attendees reported that the group helped them to [56]:

- Learn useful information
- Improve adaptation to living with pain
- Gain insights into different methods of coping with pain
- Adopt wellness behaviors
- Increase motivation
- Expand their social network

Despite positive research reports, the potential for support groups to reinforce maladaptive thoughts and behaviors does exist. Well-structured groups can help people with pain learn adaptive ways of coping from fellow sufferers better than from family members or professionals [56]. Support groups that follow the philosophy and guidelines of the American Chronic Pain Association (ACPA) do safeguard against that potential drawback. These groups take the following pledge:

- We do not dwell on physical symptoms of pain.
- We focus on abilities, not disabilities.
- We recognize and talk freely about our feelings about pain and its control over our lives.
- We do not make judgments. Group discussions are confidential.
- We use relaxation exercises to help ease the tension that increases pain and redirect attention away from our pain and suffering.
- We demonstrate mild stretching exercises and encourage you to do them daily, if your doctor approves.
- We set realistic goals and evaluate them weekly. This helps members to see that their desires can be achieved, one step at a time.
- We recognize our basic rights, including the right to make mistakes, the right to say no, and the right to ask questions.

The ACPA Web site (http://www.theacpa.org) has a directory to help locate affiliated support groups, and also can be reached by telephone at 1-800-533-3231 for more information.

Volunteering

In patients who are unable to work, volunteering can provide benefits. A study examining the transition from patient to volunteer status noted improvements in pain, disability, and depression during training and after serving in the volunteer role, without evidence of harm [57]. Making a connection with others and restoring a sense of purpose are rewarding aspects of volunteer service.

Effective communication is the foundation upon which social interactions are based. From a nursing perspective, rapport and trust are necessary before patients can accept nursing assistance in coping. Helping patients communicate in a clear, assertive, direct manner is equally important. Sometimes, patients have difficulty communicating because they are unclear about what they want; therefore, it may be helpful to explore the patient's goals with him or her [38]. Nurses also can help a patient improve his or her ability to interact socially by enhancing self-efficacy. This is accomplished through providing encouragement, teaching self-management skills, sharing vicarious experiences of successful patients, and persuading patients to act on their own behalf [58].

> **GENERAL: MANAGING FLARE-UPS**
>
> Patients may use a combination of nondrug techniques, depending on the degree of pain at any given time. On good days, pain relief and wellness behaviors (i.e., diet, exercise, relaxation, and pacing) that prevent flare-ups can be used. With mild flare-ups, curtailing activity, applying heat or cold, using massage, imagery, energy work, and problem-solving are appropriate. During major flare-ups, additional activities with high distraction value, communication skills, and problem-solving often help.

Conclusion

By themselves, conventional medical and CAM approaches have limits to their safety or efficacy. Combined they can provide a more comprehensive approach. Promoting comfort and healing is always possible, even when complete pain relief is not. An integrated approach allows nurses to restore health, joy, functioning, and a sense of purpose despite severe or persistent pain.

8 Advanced Techniques and Technologies for Pain Control

Adv. Tech.

CHAPTER 8

Advanced Techniques and Technologies for Pain Control

This chapter will review the safe, effective use of common technology-assisted analgesia methods. Nonoperative and minimally invasive procedures used to control pain also are described and conclude with emerging innovations.

Technology-Assisted Analgesia

Technology-assisted analgesia delivers medication in a way that minimizes analgesic gaps and side effects. To promote safety, it is advised that organizations using these technologies provide the following best-practice elements [1]:

- Written and verbal education of patients and family members
- Written and verbal education of professionals, with documented competency
- Pocket safety cards and periodic reeducation of professionals
- Intranet access to policies and guidelines
- Electronic systems for order entry, dispensing, and medication administration
  - Smart-pump technologies with drug-specific libraries and protocols
  - Bar-coded labels
  - Limited need to bypass safety features (work-arounds)
- Limited choices of medications and drug concentrations available
- Real-time, ongoing monitoring and quality improvement systems

Despite these enhancements, technically proficient, astute nursing care is the key factor ensuring the safety and efficacy of these devices. Nurses are responsible for:

- Monitoring patient responses
- Ensuring correct pump settings
- Ensuring the integrity of the system during each shift
- Ensuring accuracy of drug picks and pump settings
  - Whenever bags or settings are changed
  - At change of shift
  - Whenever patients are transported

Nurses systematically check the integrity of the insertion site, dressing, and delivery system. This includes checks of:

- Catheter insertion site and dressing for fluid leakage, signs of infection, or bleeding
- Connections; assuring they are secure, without leaks or clamps obstructing flow
- Pump settings, power source, and alarms
- Labeling of medication
- Medication solution for clarity and medication container is free of cracks or leaks

The frequency of these assessments is determined by organizational policy and the patient's condition. At every transition in care (i.e., transfer between units, change of medication bag or pump settings, shift change), the responsible nurse verifies the system integrity, checks the pump settings, and assesses the patient.

Continuous IV Opioid Infusions

The IV route provides rapid and effective pain relief with predictable pharmacological effects. Depending on the drug, expect the onset of relief in 5 to 20 min and the peak of both desired and adverse effects (such as respiratory depression) within 30 min. Blood levels of most opioids stabilize between 8 and 20 hr when a continuous infusion rate is sustained. For that reason, it is best to adjust the continuous rate no more than once or twice a day for most agents.

> **ALERT**
>
> Hundreds of wrong-route errors, some fatal, occur because of misconnected tubing. Tubing errors can misdirect medications, bacteria, toxic fluids, or compressed air to vital organs. High-risk (i.e., epidural, intrathecal, arterial) catheters always should be clearly labeled indicating their route. Always administer medications and change tubing and medication bags in a well-lit environment, and always double-check pump settings before leaving the bedside. Trace a tube from the patient to connection and the medication source before starting any infusion, and during transitions in care. Never force connections that do not fit [2, 3].

Guidelines for titrating the infusion rate are as follows:
- The typical increase in the infusion rate is 25% to 50%
- A 100% increase is the maximum change at one time
- Give a bolus dose when rate is increased to shorten time to steady state
- Assess patient within 30 min after a bolus and/or a rate increase
- Reassess pain, sedation, and breathing at least every 4 hr, according to policy

Other Considerations

Satisfactory respiratory rate and pain level are considered the endpoints of therapy, so even if a patient is itching or has low-blood pressure, continuous infusion rates can be increased as long as respiratory rate is satisfactory and pain level is unacceptable.

- Patients on continuous opioid infusions will likely develop constipation, so a bowel regimen is advised (see Chapter 6).
- In patients who lose IV access, infusions can be continued using the subcutaneous (SQ) route, although drug concentrations may need to be adjusted to accommodate lower flow rates (< 3 mL/hr) appropriate for SQ infusions.
- In dying patients, when kidneys fail then medications may need adjustment to prevent agitation, delirium, and myoclonus resulting from metabolite accumulation [6].

The nurse observes and documents the pattern of analgesic use and the patient's response. See Table 8–1 for details of the assessments and documentation required.

Patient-Controlled Analgesia

Patient-controlled analgesia (PCA) uses technology that permits patients to self-administer pain medicine as needed. Devices can administer PCA by various routes (i.e., oral, SQ, epidural, intrathecal), but the IV route is most common. Ideally, PCA avoids side effects by allowing patients to self-administer the smallest, effective dose. Locking mechanisms prevent unauthorized access to excessive opioid doses.

Table 8–1 Assessment and Monitoring Required for Technology-Assisted Analgesia

	CONTINUOUS IV OPIOID INFUSION	PATIENT-CONTROLLED IV ANALGESIA	SPINAL ANALGESIA	PERINEURAL ANALGESIA
Kinetic Advantage	Avoids first pass through liver	Avoids first pass, medication used only when needed	Avoids first pass and plasma proteins, blood-brain barrier	Avoids first pass, plasma proteins, blood–brain barrier
Benefits	Rapid onset, predictable effects, ease of titration	Rapid onset, predictable effects, ease of titration, patient involvement in care Often less medicine used	Superior analgesia Lower GI side effects, lower risk of sedation, respiratory depression	Superior analgesia Lower GI side effects, lower risk of sedation, respiratory depression
Most Common Adverse Events	Nausea, vomiting, pruritus, constipation	Nausea, vomiting, pruritus, constipation	Pruritus, nausea, sensory/motor block, orthostasis	Sensory/motor block
Most Serious Adverse Event	Somnolence, respiratory depression, infection/sepsis	Somnolence, respiratory depression, infection/sepsis	Infection (abscess, meningitis, etc), hemorrhage (hematoma), paralysis, toxicity	Infection, hemorrhage, nerve damage, systemic toxicity
Route-Specific Monitoring	Respiratory rate, sedation, pain level Some patients may have O_2 levels or CO_2 levels monitored	Patient ability to understand and operate device Pattern of use to anticipate analgesic need when changing to different form of therapy Same as IV opioid infusion	Vital signs, sedation, sensory/motor (new worsening or unilateral) deficit, toxicity, risk of falling before ambulating	Falls risk Motor weakness Vital signs (e.g., fever, respiration, orthostasis), sedation, toxicity Monitor for signs of complications (other than pain)

	CONTINUOUS IV OPIOID INFUSION	PATIENT-CONTROLLED IV ANALGESIA	SPINAL ANALGESIA	PERINEURAL ANALGESIA
Table 8–1 Assessment and Monitoring Required for Technology-Assisted Analgesia—cont'd				
Safety Precautions	Double-check pump settings, connections, IV site	Double-check pump settings, connections, IV site	Double-check pump settings, label connections, color-coded tubes	Fall precautions Double-check pump settings, label connections Use preservative-free solution only

The foundational safety principles of PCA therapy are careful patient selection, effective education, accurate device programming, and vigilant monitoring. Each organization details and monitors its systems for ordering, stocking, and labeling medications for PCA therapy to minimize the risk of errors. Despite many safety features built into the technology and precautions written in policies, one-half of all opioid-related adverse events occur while patients are using PCA technology [1, 8].

PCA-by-proxy (doses activated by someone other than the patient) is particularly risky [9]. This practice overrides the inherent safety assumption that a patient who is at risk of imminent overdose is too sedated to operate the device. In unique circumstances, someone other than the patient may be required to activate the device. To do this safely, strict training, procedures, and monitoring guidelines must be followed [10].

COACH CONSULT

PCA can be delivered by a variety of routes. IV and epidural forms are the most common route of analgesia delivery. Devices now permit PCA therapy via regional, oral, intranasal, and transdermal routes. Ideal systems are easy to use, permit self-titration with safeguards preventing programming errors and patient overdose [7].

Devices used for PCA therapy generally have more than one way of delivering medication. There is a clinician-activated bolus dose, typically used as a "loading dose" at the beginning of therapy; the patient-activated PCA dose; and a basal-rate feature that can deliver a continuous infusion independent of either a clinician or patient-activated dose [11]. For most opioid-naïve patients with acute pain, a basal rate is *not* included in the initial order. A basal rate increases the risk of respiratory depression and should *not* be used in at-risk patients, including those who:

- Are opioid naïve
- Have a history of sleep apnea (unless wearing CPAP*)
- Are markedly obese (BMI** > 40)
- Have had thoracic, neck, or upper-abdominal surgery or trauma (risk of hypoventilation)
- Have renal insufficiency
- Are pediatric or elderly patients
- Are in an unmonitored environment
- Have concurrent diseases or drugs that affect breathing

Good candidates for the basal-rate feature are opioid-tolerant patients who have an established daily analgesic requirement.

The basic components of a PCA order include the following:

- Incremental dose that the patient may self-administer by activating the demand button
- Lockout interval: the time period between doses when no additional dose is available
- The maximum safe limit, typically ordered as a 1-hr limit

Additional optional parts of a PCA order may include:

- Bolus dose: activated by the nurse at the start of therapy or for breakthrough pain
- Titration range for the nurse to adjust the patient's demand (incremental) dose
- Basal rate for providing a continuous infusion of opioid

The nurse observes and documents the pattern of analgesic use and the patient's response. See Table 8–1 for details of the safety precautions and monitoring required.

Perineural Analgesia

Continuous perineural analgesia (CPA) entails infusing a local anesthetic adjacent to relevant nerves that are signaling the patient's pain. The

---

* CPAP is a continuous positive airway pressure device.
** BMI is a Body Mass Index calculation of weight relative to height.

NURSE-TO-NURSE TIP

The patient's emotional state is often overlooked as a barrier to effective PCA therapy. Patients may have the understanding, dexterity, and strength necessary to operate the device but still refrain out of fear of becoming overdosed or addicted. Reassure the patient the PCA doses are a fraction of what they would receive in a standard injection. Prompt the patient to activate the PCA device every 10 to 15 min until pain is controlled.

advantages of these regional approaches include superior pain control without opioid-associated side effects [12]. CPA can expedite rehabilitative efforts. However, local anesthetics do cause problems that may slow recovery. These include:

- Motor block may produce weakness or inability to exercise
- Sympathetic block may produce low-blood pressure, including orthostatic changes
- Sympathetic and motor blocks combined may increase risk of falling
- Lack of pain may lead to delayed identification of complications

Although CPA may result in shortened length of stay, true long-term benefits demand high-efficiency teamwork to achieve the optimal balance between analgesia and functioning. This may require scheduled dose reductions or interruptions of therapy a few hours before physical therapy, and an effective fall prevention program.

The nurse observes and documents the local, regional and systemic effects of the medications (see Table 8–1). Stop the infusion and inform the medical provider if any of the following occur:

- Symptoms suggestive of systemic (local anesthetic) toxicity:
  - *Early signs:* thick tongue sensation, metallic or weird taste in mouth, numbness around lips, the feeling of a fuzzy head, or ringing in the ears
  - *Late signs:* (rare) seizures, cardiac arrhythmias, or cardiac arrest
- Excessive leakage, redness, drainage, or pain at insertion site
- Occlusion of the infusion
- Significant changes in vital signs
- Unusual or high-intensity pain

A variety of approaches are used based on the location and nature of pain. Scalene blocks for shoulder pain, femoral blocks for leg pain, and paravertebral blocks for thoracic pain are the most common CPA types (see Table 8–2).

Table 8–2 Common Types of Continuous Perineural Analgesia Blocks

TYPE	INDICATIONS	ADVERSE EFFECTS	COMMENTS
Interscalene	Shoulder, arm, or hand surgery Complex Regional Pain Syndrome	Abnormal (hot, heavy) or numb sensation of arm or hand Horner's syndrome, hoarseness, swallowing difficulty Pneumothorax (rare)	Do not lay patient flat (elevate head of bed ≥30°) NPO until ability to swallow safely is established.
Femoral	Major knee or lower extremity surgery	Leg weakness, urinary retention	Evaluate risk of falling before ambulation
Paravertebral	Thoracic or breast surgery	Unilateral or bilateral numbness, hypotension, urinary retention Bradycardia or pneumothorax (rare)	Two catheters may be placed. May be used with PCA technology. Evaluate risk of falling before ambulation.

ALERT

Local anesthetics, such as bupivacaine (Marcaine) and ropivacaine (Naropin) commonly are used for perineural infusions because of the relatively long duration of desired actions. Problems with short-term neurotoxicity and cardiotoxicity have long been known, with numb lips, thick tongue, or metallic taste serving as an early warning sign. Emerging evidence suggests that these local anesthetics

Continued

Intraspinal Analgesia

The administration of analgesics into the epidural or intrathecal (subarachnoid) space (Fig. 8–1), is generally safer and more efficacious than IV analgesia. Analgesics are delivered in close proximity to the nerve targets (opioid receptors, sodium channels). This route bypasses plasma proteins, hepatic circulation, the blood-brain barrier, and other factors that lower the amount of free drug available to receptors. Thus, smaller doses are required, with fewer systemic effects. Another distinguishing feature is that intraspinal infusions can be stopped, left in place for minutes or hours, and restarted without concerns about clotting off the catheter. Therapy can be delivered in the following ways:

- Bolus doses, either one-time or intermittent
- Continuous infusion
- Combination of continuous infusion plus intermittent bolus doses

For percutaneous approaches, intraspinal analgesia is typically limited to no longer than a few days. For long-term therapy, implanted devices with internal pumps and tunneled catheters are available.

The nurse observes and documents the desired effects and provides ongoing, vigilant monitoring for uncommon but catastrophic complications, such as spinal infection or hematoma (see Table 8–1). All medications are preservative free, because preservatives may be toxic to nerves.

Epidural Analgesia

The epidural route is most commonly used for short-term analgesia because of the lower risk of infection and headache compared with the intrathecal route. The epidural space is a fatty and highly vascular area separated from the spinal cord by the dura mater. Fat-soluble medications, such as fentanyl, have limited spread in the epidural space and are readily absorbed into the bloodstream [14]. As a result, epidural fentanyl may have more opioid-related side effects than other epidural drugs.

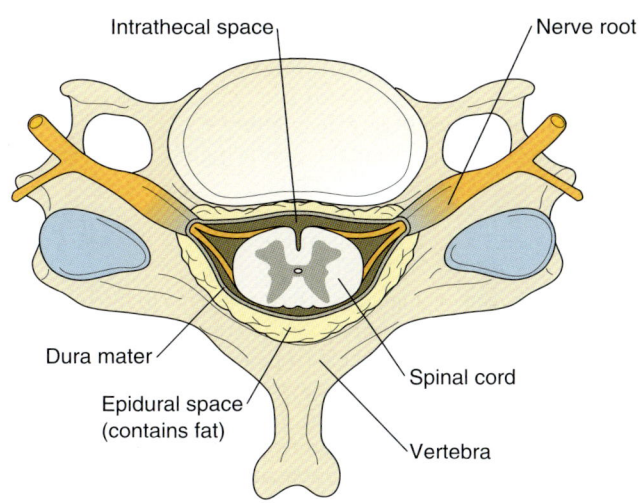

F I G U R E 8 – 1 : Spinal anatomy: epidural and intrathecal spaces. Intrathecal space contains cerebrospinal fluid and the spinal cord and is separated from the epidural space by the protective dura mater.

In contrast, water-soluble drugs, such as morphine have a good "volume column spread" with negligible uptake into fat cells and the bloodstream. This spread within the epidural space provides a broad band of analgesic coverage with greater potency and longer duration of action compared with parenteral morphine. However, epidural morphine causes more itching and urinary retention than IV morphine. Therefore, epidural hydromorphone (Dilaudid), with fewer side effects with a good band of analgesic coverage often is used instead of morphine.

Most often, an epidural is a continuous infusion, perhaps with patient-controlled capabilities added [15]. A local anesthetic (e.g., bupivacaine) is at least one of the ingredients infused in most cases. Although few serious side effects are seen with local anesthetics, patients may be at increased risk for falling [10]. A single epidural bolus typically works within 30 min and lasts for up to 6 hr, therefore, patients are monitored until 4 to 6 hr after the infusion is stopped [16]. A notable exception is DepoDur, which is a controlled-release epidural morphine bolus that lasts for 48 hr [17].

Nursing care of patients with spinal anesthesia includes testing sensory and motor function. A new, unilateral, or progressive deficit may be a sign of complications (e.g., hematoma or abscess) or a warning that the patient has an elevated risk of injury (e.g., falls, burns). To assess sensory function, swipe a wet alcohol swab in areas representing key dermatomes bilaterally [14, 15]. Record the patient's response as normal, diminished, or absent.

The following areas represent key dermatomes:

C_8 = Little Finger L_1 = Medial Upper Thigh/Groin
T_4 = Nipple L_2 = Medial Thigh
T_6 = Xiphoid L_3 = Medial Knee
T_{10} = Naval L_4 = Medial Ankle
T_{12} = Pubis L_5 = Dorsal Foot

Motor Function is best evaluated by asking patients to move their toes and feet, then ask them (unless contraindicated) to raise their feet off the bed and bring their knees up toward the chest (repeated against resistance if unimpaired). Motor function is evaluated for symmetry and rated on a 0-to-5 scale:

0. No movement—no contraction
1. Muscle flicker but no movement
2. Moves on bed (horizontal), not against gravity
3. Moves against gravity, not resistance
4. Moves against some examiner resistance
5. Normal strength

Intrathecal Analgesia

Intrathecal administration delivers medication directly into the cerebrospinal fluid (CSF) (Box 8–1).

When drugs are delivered via the intrathecal route, respiratory depression may be delayed. Medication leaves the spinal (pain-blocking) receptors and circulates to the brain to be eliminated via the subarachnoid plexus [19, 20]. During this process, the drug may rebind to opioid receptors in the brain that regulate respiratory rate.

Intrathecal anesthesia may be administered as a one-time dose, or temporary percutaneous catheters may deliver infusions for hours or days [18]. Prolonged intrathecal analgesia may be delivered using a tunneled catheter and implanted pump system. Implanted intrathecal analgesia systems are highly effective, but controversial [19] because:

- Surgical implantation of the device carries risks
- Initial and maintenance costs are high
- Nearly a quarter of patients require surgery to correct technical problems [20, 21]
- Side effects include endocrine and urinary dysfunction, granulomas, and edema
- Functional improvement is not consistently realized [19, 20]

Although only morphine, ziconotide, and baclofen (antispasmotic) have U.S. Food and Drug Administration (FDA) approval for intrathecal therapy, a variety of other drugs are used off-label. Ziconotide is a treatment

> **ALERT** ❗
>
> Formation of a hematoma or abscess is a rare but catastrophic complication of spinal analgesia. Progressive sensory/motor block and low-back pain, with or without a fever are hallmark signs. Vigilant monitoring for all patients with spinal analgesia, at least every 4 hr, is needed. When problems are suspected, medical evaluation, including magnetic resonance imaging (MRI), with possible emergency decompression surgery must be completed within 8 hr of symptom onset to minimize the risk of persistent paralysis.

Box 8–1 Comparison of Delivery Routes

The *spinal* route is the most effective for drug delivery. By the *oral* route, incomplete absorption and the first pass through the liver results in delivery of only a small portion of the administered drug to systemic circulation. *IV* drugs become bound to plasma proteins or tissue stores throughout the body. *Epidural* drugs only partially diffuse to the spinal cord, while *intrathecal* drugs bathe the spinal cord adjacent to the infusion site. Relative potencies for morphine by route are [18] as follows:

300 mg oral = 100 mg IV = 10 mg epidural = 1 mg intrathecal

of last resort. On average, patients achieve a 30% reduction in pain; however toxicity and unacceptable side effects limit its usefulness for most patients [22, 23].

Postimplantation complications include disconnection, breakage, and obstruction of the catheter; cerebrospinal fluid leaks; overdose; granuloma formation at the catheter tip; and seroma formation or infection at the pump pouch. Care of patients with implanted systems is done in pain specialty clinics. It is useful to know the resources available in your community to help patients with this technology, or in the event out-of-town patients present with pump-related needs.

Invasive Procedures

When systemic analgesics are contraindicated or problematic, well-selected invasive procedures can reduce or eliminate pain and improve functioning and quality of life. Table 8–3 describes the most common invasive techniques. Interventional approaches increasingly are being used to identify and quiet "pain generators." Sometimes these techniques produce profound results and eliminate the need for systemic analgesics; more often they provide partial, temporary relief. Even with optimum technique, bleeding, infection, or embolism can occur. Therefore asepsis, vigilant monitoring, and access to resuscitative equipment are needed.

Nurses may be involved with care coordination, providing patients with information needed for informed consent, and providing direct care before, during, or after these interventions. A basic understanding of common interventional options (Table 8–3), the typical postprocedural course, and related nursing care requirements are reviewed here.

Trigger Point Injections

Injecting palpable, tender, taut bands of muscle is common in general and specialty practices. Trigger points are small irritable "knots" in the muscle and fascia that irritate or entrap nerves, producing referred or radiating pain. Injection may be with saline or local anesthetic alone, followed by stretching or using myofascial manipulation to release the spasm. Rarely, the anesthetic is mistakenly infused into a blood vessel causing an immediate medical emergency demanding nursing attention. More commonly, the only side effect is pain at the injection site. Muscles can become damaged. Skin atrophy, hypopigmentation, and dimpling at the site can occur if steroids are used. Local tissue damage can

Table 8–3 Invasive Procedures for Managing Pain

PROCEDURE	DESCRIPTION	INDICATIONS	COMPLICATIONS
Epidural Steroids	Inject steroids to cut inflammation from disk, nerve root, or other source	Radiculopathy spinal stenosis, herniated disk, nerve root tumor	Back pain, hypertension, hyperglycemia, spinal headache, epidural hematoma or abscess, meningitis, nerve injury
Facet Injections	Inject local anesthetic or steroid into facet joint	Neck/back pain Facet arthritis	Infection, radicular pain, intrathecal injection, nerve block/injury from errant needle placement
Intradiscal Electrothermal Annuloplasty	Fluoroscopy-guided catheter heats and treats herniated disk	Disk-related, low-back pain Analgesic failure	Infection, discitis, catheter breaks, bone necrosis, paralysis, incontinence
Intrathecal Opioid Pump	Percutaneous or implanted medication-infusion device	Severe pain responsive to opioid, when treatment is limited by side effects	Infection, hematoma, granuloma formation, catheter breaks, spinal or nerve injury, CSF leaks, pump complications
Percutaneous Nucleoplasty	Guided needle heats disk by radio waves	Herniated disk, low-back pain	Infection, catheter breaks, nerve injury
Radiofrequency Lesion	Radio-wave heat damages nerves or pain-producing tissue	Diagnostic block identifies nerve producing pain	Vertigo, sensory change, pain, pneumothorax, nerve damage, bleeding, infection, spasm
Sacroiliac Joint Injections	Local anesthetic injected under fluoroscopic guidance	Sacroiliac trauma, arthritis, strain, sciatica pattern	Infection, bleeding, flare of back pain

Continued

Table 8–3 Invasive Procedures for Managing Pain—cont'd

PROCEDURE	DESCRIPTION	INDICATIONS	COMPLICATIONS
Spinal Cord Stimulators	Impulses stimulate inhibitory nerves	Treatment failure, severe pain, ischemic pain	Bleeding, infection, migration or breakage of leads
Sympathetic Blocks: Stellate Ganglion, Celiac Plexus, Lumbar, etc.	Block sympathetic chains involved in pain transmission or amplification	Visceral pain, ischemic pain	Infection, intravascular injection, bleeding, tissue and organ damage
Trigger Point Injection	Inject taut, tender muscle band with local anesthetic	Myofascial pain done before physical therapy treatment	Infection, bleeding, nerve injury, muscle atrophy, skin color loss
Vertebroplasty/ Kyphoplasty	Inject cement into broken vertebrae	Vertebral compression fracture	Infection, injury, cement leak, pulmonary emboli

occur if a high volume of concentrated local anesthetic is used. The area injected often is tender for a couple of days, which is treated with topical nondrug method (e.g., ice or massage) and stretching.

Intradiscal Electrothermal Therapy

With intradiscal electrothermal therapy (IDET), treatment of a herniated or degenerated intervertebral disk is accomplished by applying electrothermal (or radiofrequency) energy for 10 to 15 min. Heat damages sensitive nerves and alters collagen fibers within the disk responsible for inflammation or pain. Pain relief begins within a few days and lasts up to 6 months following the procedure. The long-term risks and benefits of this procedure are unclear, and the Centers for Medicare & Medicaid Services decided to stop reimbursing for these procedures. Compared with other options for a herniated or degenerated disk, this has lower risk of complications and an easier rehabilitation phase. After the procedure, nurses monitor vital signs and for any sensory/motor or bowel/bladder dysfunction.

Artificial Disk Replacement

Prosthetic joints have long been available for knees and hips; and now an option exists for those with degenerative disk disease. The prosthetic disk removes the presumed (1 level) source of pain while preserving range of motion and spinal stability. The relative novelty of this technology makes it unclear what long-term risks and benefits can be expected; however, nurses should watch for sudden pain, asymmetry, and neurological dysfunction that would indicate the prosthesis has slipped out of place.

Percutaneous Coblation Nucleoplasty

Minimally invasive disk decompression is considered safest when bipolar radiofrequency (coblation) procedures are used. The technique dissolves target tissue, creates a series of channels, and/or reduces the volume of hypertrophied tissues while minimizing damage to surrounding, healthy cells. With this minimally invasive approach, there are fewer complications and expedited recovery times, with some patients returning to work in a week. After the procedure, nurses monitor vital signs and for any sensory/motor or bowel/bladder dysfunction. Any itching, insertion site soreness, muscle spasms, nausea, or vomiting are treated symptomatically after the procedure.

Interspinous Spacer Devices

A device, such as the X-Stop, used for spinal stenosis, may be surgically implanted between the interspinous processes to widen the space between vertebrae and limit painful extension of the spine. It is placed between the spinal processes at the level of stenosis using local anesthesia on an outpatient basis. Given a small incision, no bone or soft-tissue removal and no manipulation of nerves or the spinal cord; this procedure is considered relatively safe with a short convalescence period. Patients often feel better immediately after the procedure, but are warned to avoid sports, heavy lifting, stair climbing, or bending backward for the first several weeks to prevent stress fractures or device failure.

Vertebroplasty or Kyphoplasty

Vertebral fractures are a common cause of back pain in older adults, often secondary to osteoporosis. To prevent the pulmonary and gastrointestinal (GI) morbidity that occurs when severe pain cannot be managed by conservative methods, vertebroplasty and kyphoplasty may be used. In vertebroplasty, bone cement is injected through a hollow needle into the fractured bone. In kyphoplasty, balloons (one on each side) are inserted into the vertebrae, which are inflated to restore the height and shape of the vertebra. The balloons then are removed and cement is injected into the cavity created by the balloons. Whereas both relieve pain, kyphoplasty restores vertebral height and shape. About 5% of patients have serious complications, the most catastrophic of which are paraplegia, stroke, or pulmonary embolism related to cement leakage. Although more expensive; kyphoplasty may be the better of these procedures because of better restoration of vertebral height and less risk of cement leakage.

Postoperative care requirements involve monitoring patients during their emergence from conscious sedation, observing for signs of infection, and neurological deficits suggestive of complications.

Epidural Steroid Injections

Epidural steroids are indicated for back pain that radiates to leg pain (sciatica) or its counterpart affecting the arm (cervical brachialgia). These radiculopathies can be due to disk-induced nerve irritation, spinal stenosis, or nerve entrapment. A bolus of steroid is placed at the nerve root (transforaminal; see Box 8–2 for dangers), or between the dura and the spine (interlaminar) at the affected level or from below via a caudal approach. During the procedure, the patient is awake, but may be sedated, so he or she can provide feedback to the nurse about sensations of pain or numbness. Sterile technique is strictly adhered to and masks are worn to reduce the rate of infection. Patients are monitored for an hour before being discharged, and they are informed to expect pain at the injection site for a couple of days. The effects of the local anesthetic are immediate, but wear off quickly, as the effects of the steroid take a few days to achieve their pain-relieving benefit. Controversies aside (see Box 8–3), nurses often assist with the positioning and care of the patient, before, during, and after the procedure.

Facet (Zygapophyseal) Joint Blocks

Facet joints stabilize the vertebrae and permit bending and twisting of the back. Although they are thought to be a common source of pain, no

---

Box 8–2 **Transforaminal Dangers**

Transforaminal epidural injections are considered precise and effective. However, dozens of devastating brain and spinal injuries, including 12 deaths, have been reported from this procedure. Cervical injections are more risky than those involving the lumbar region. Microcrystals in corticosteroids, such as methylprednisolone (e.g., Medrol or Solu-Medrol), injected into microvasculature are the presumed culprit. As a precaution, interventionists are switching to less effective water-soluble steroids, such as dexamethasone (e.g., Decaron, Dexasone) and using digital subtraction angiography to ensure microembolization does not occur [24].

Nurses should be familiar with controversies surrounding epidural steroid injection (ESI) to guide their "coordination of care" or "patient education and counseling" roles. First, the technique may be done blind or be guided by radiographic equipment. Radiographic guidance targeting identifiable defects are preferred, as 85% of "blind" techniques (placing needles based on anatomic landmarks) miss their target, accounting for wide variations in reported response rates by that method [19, 20]. Concern has been raised that many patients referred for ESI lack the clear indication of acute radicular pain known to benefit from the procedure [20, 21]. Controversies about the most effective approach, midline (interlaminar) versus lateral (transforaminal), exist. The more precise transforaminal approach is preferred for greater efficacy, unless riskier cervical injections are needed. The caudal approach passes through the tailbone and is considered best where scar tissue may be responsible for the symptoms.

clinical or radiographic assessments can confirm this assumption. Repeated diagnostic blocks are the only means by which the source of a patient's pain can be traced to their facet joints. Injection of corticosteroid into the facet joints is problem-prone, and the practice largely has been replaced by blocking the "medial branch" nerve that innervates the joints. Because successful medial branch blocks provide only several hours of relief at best [25], they are considered diagnostic. Two or more successful blocks are needed for patients to be considered candidates for radiofrequency lesions that provide longer-term relief [26].

Neurolysis (Nerve-Deadening) Procedures

When a diagnostic nerve block is successful at providing temporary symptomatic relief, then neurolytic approaches are offered to achieve prolonged relief. In the past, alcohol or phenol was used to deaden nerves but they caused pain problems of their own. In rare situations, surgical interventions cut nerves in the spinal cord or brain. These procedures largely have been replaced by localized heating (i.e., radiofrequency lesioning) or freezing (i.e., cryoanalagesia) techniques.

First the specific sensory nerve is isolated, followed by the heating or freezing tip that creates the lesion. Motor responses are not desired and the patient should report "tingling" or "buzzing," not pain. Pain may flare after the procedure for hours or days, before pain relief improves over several days to weeks. Transient numbness is expected, but fever, persistent numbness, weakness, or paralysis must be reported and evaluated in an expedient fashion.

Sympathetic Nerve Blocks

The way that a sympathetic nerve abnormality can generate, prolong, and spread pain was described in Chapter 3 on physiology. Blocking these sympathetic pain generators can be approached from IV, intraspinal, or regional approaches. Although hypotension is expected with many sympathetic blocks, other block-specific effects should be anticipated. Major ganglia within the sympathetic chain targeted, including:

- Stellate ganglion block for pain in head or neck
- Thoracic ganglia blocks for arm pain
- Splanchnic block for upper abdominal visceral pain
- Celiac plexus block for abdominal visceral pain (often pancreatic)
- Hypogastric plexus block for lower abdominal and pelvic visceral pain
- Lumbar sympathetic ganglia block for leg pain

The blocks are usually accomplished with a local anesthetic bolus, however alpha-adrenergic blockers (i.e., clonidine, phenoxybenzamine) and sympatholytic agents (guanethidine, reserpine) also are used alone or in combination. Neurolysis (e.g., radiofrequency denervation) of sympathetic ganglia may give more lasting effects, but unfortunately the benefits are unpredictable and the potential risks of vascular problems are added to those of other nerve blocks. Monitoring for bleeding, infection, and hemodynamic changes is warranted.

Electrical Nerve Stimulation

Electrical stimulation suppresses sympathetic nervous system activity, thereby promoting arterial circulation and reducing ischemic pain. It also is believed to stimulate the production of endorphins and other pain suppressing neurotransmitters. Patients are awake during the implantation procedures to help the interventionist place the electrodes where they provide the greatest coverage. *Peripheral nerve stimulation* is effective for

 NURSE-TO-NURSE TIP

A Bier block (IV regional sympatholysis) helps diagnose sympathetically maintained pain. First a tourniquet isolates the affected limb from systemic circulation before guanethidine is injected. Nurses often are called upon to monitor the patient and manage the tourniquet release part of the procedure that begins 20 min after blood flow is restricted. Cautious monitoring of pressure settings and slow tourniquet release at specified intervals are needed. Nasal congestion, hypotension, and dysrhythmias may occur, suggesting the tourniquet release may need to be slowed.

some types of painful peripheral neuropathies, with a fascia graft used to anchor the electrode in place. *Deep-brain stimulation* or *electroconvulsive therapy (ECT)* for pain have anecdotal evidence of effectiveness for severe central neuropathic pain; but these are largely last-line options and experimental. *Spinal cord stimulation* (*SCS*) involves the implantation of electrodes into the spinal column that corresponds to the area of severe persistent pain. Although serious complications are rare, they can be disastrous causing additional pain, neurologic injury, and the need for delicate spinal surgery [27]. Immediately after surgery, nurses monitor patients for adverse effects and medicate them for surgical site pain, chronic pain, and muscle spasm.

Nurses monitor vital signs, and for evidence of neurological deficits, hemorrhage, or infection. Patients must be educated about strict activity restriction and hygiene that is needed in the postoperative period to prevent infection, migration, or damage to the system. These patients need to wear Medic Alert bracelets, and may need periodic adjustments if they develop uncomfortable jolting or shocklike sensations [28].

Trends and Future Assumptions

Basic research in recent years has identified dozens of therapeutic targets resulting in the emergence of new classes of pain relievers now in development. The global market for pain relief is expected to grow by 25% through 2014, and nonopioids are expected to make up a major portion of this market [29]. New drug-delivery systems include:

- Using electrical currents (iontophoresis) to transport drugs across the skin
- Abuse-deterrent formulas and packaging that curtails opioid abuse or diversion

Some new medications use a two-drug combination either to make nerves more receptive to the active drug or to help release the active drug from implanted depots when needed. Some new products will have a duration measured weeks rather than hours. Gene therapy uses a deactivated version of herpes simplex virus with a high affinity for nerve cells to deliver genes that will stimulate endogenous opioid production for 3 months or longer [30].

There will be an expanded use of currently available nondrug technologies including:

- Low-level lasers [31–34]
- Noninvasive transcranial electrical stimulation techniques [35]
- Mirror-box therapy and virtual reality [36, 37]

ON THE HORIZON

An innovative iontophoretic transdermal system provides on-demand delivery of 45 mcg fentanyl available every 10 min. Over 24 hr, the device will deliver a maximum of 80 doses. The FDA approved this device in 2007, but marketing and distribution have been stalled due to unforeseen technical and disposal concerns. Enthusiasts believe this system will replace IV PCA someday, but system refinements are needed.

As patients become more technologically savvy, electronic devices will increasingly be used to educate patients, monitor their progress, and facilitate communication with professionals. The use of electronic pain diaries in research and clinical practice is already providing patients and caregivers with real-time information organized in a way that supports decisions about optimal treatment strategies [38]. Web-based therapies also will expand in number and scope [39].

Despite the anticipated development of technologies, opportunities for promoting the use of available safe, effective, pain-relieving technologies extend from the bedside to the boardroom. Many helpful, cost-effective approaches to treating pain have been abandoned, in part because the reimbursement structure, not patient need, often drives health-care decisions. For example, unimodal, interventional pain programs that provide limited, temporary relief to carefully selected patients have flourished because reimbursement dollars have supported their growth. Meanwhile, more effective multidisciplinary, multimodal treatment programs, or cognitive-behavior programs that can be led by nurses, have been closed because they are noncovered, despite evidence of cost-effectiveness [40, 41]. Nurses are in a key position to help replace the barriers of unrealistic fear and mistaken belief about available treatments by facilitating processes that support informed decision making and maintenance of a patient-centered focus.

9 Controlling Pain in Specific Patient Populations

Special Pop.

CHAPTER 9

Controlling Pain in Specific Patient Populations

Each year, 50 million Americans have pain after surgery [1], and at least 75 million more are living with painful disorders, such as cancer, sickle cell anemia, back pain, or arthritis [2–5]. About one-half of patients with pain remain undertreated. This is true for newborns [6], children, and other special populations, such as cancer patients and the elderly. This chapter highlights population-specific challenges, and "pearls" to help the nurse individualize care across the life span and address diagnoses associated with challenging forms of pain.

Maternal Pain Relief

During Pregnancy

The developing fetus is vulnerable to harmful effects of medicine. Therefore throughout pregnancy, labor, and delivery, the focus is on pain prevention and using nondrug relief techniques. Pregnant women most often experience mild or moderate pain located in the abdomen or back and related to stretching ligaments, pressure from the growing uterus, gastrointestinal (GI) discomforts, uterine cramping, or Braxton Hicks contractions. The following interventions often bring relief:

- Position changes
- Rest
- Distraction
- Gentle massage

Additional interventions are listed in Box 9–1. Note that severe pain is uncommon during pregnancy and warrants emergency evaluation before any medication is taken.

199

Use of Analgesics During Pregnancy

If analgesics are needed during pregnancy, acetaminophen is the best choice. Aspirin and other NSAIDs are generally avoided. In situations in which acetaminophen cannot be given and an NSAID is needed early in pregnancy, ibuprofen or naproxen may be the best alternatives. The danger of NSAIDs during the first 2 trimesters is unclear; however, indomethacin has been associated with fetal brain and intestinal anomalies [8].

Late in pregnancy, NSAIDs are contraindicated as they may cause:

- Bleeding in neonate and mother
- Premature closure of ductus arteriosus
- Decreased fetal urine output, and neonatal renal impairment
- Neonatal pulmonary hypertension
- Decreased amniotic fluid volume (oligohy-dramnios)

ALERT

Although NSAIDs can suppress implantation at conception and cause a host of third-trimester problems, they are not absolutely contraindicated during pregnancy. Adjuvant drugs for neuropathic pain, such as valproic acid and amitriptyline, can cause birth defects and are avoided in women who are or may be pregnant. Misoprostol that is added to some NSAIDs to prevent stomach ulcers causes severe enough contractions to terminate pregnancy and is contraindicated in women who are or may become pregnant.

Opioids generally are considered safe if used briefly for severe acute pain. Mothers who take opioids throughout pregnancy usually bear small babies (i.e., weight and length) who develop neonatal abstinence syndrome 24 to 48 hr after birth. These neonates need opioid tapering to pre-vent associated GI, respiratory, and neurologic problems.

Use of Analgesics During Labor and Delivery

Opioids administered during labor and delivery are considered safe, but they are reserved until the late stages of labor to minimize the neonate's exposure to the respiratory depressant effects. Fat-soluble opioids, such as fentanyl are more readily transferred to the baby than are water-soluble drugs, such as morphine. Epidural or spinal analgesia and anesthetic blocks during labor reduce the baby's drug exposure and produce superior analgesia for the mother. When respiratory depression occurs in the newborn, a naloxone infusion is typically needed for a few hours until those effects wear off.

Use of Postpartum Analgesics

Postpartum maternal analgesia use can affect the breastfed baby. Nonopioids are safe because less than 1% of the medication is transferred to the baby. Low-dose opioids also are considered safe, although the U.S. Food and Drug Administration (FDA) warns against the use of codeine by breastfeeding women [11]. Some women are ultrarapid metabolizers of codeine, producing a rapid, dangerous spike in opioid concentration in breast milk.

Neonatal Pain and Its Relief

All of the elements necessary for pain are present in newborns, regardless of their gestational age [12]. An overabundance of nerves, combined with a robust inflammatory response, rapid (pain-amplifying) sensitization, neuroplasticity, and immature inhibitory nerves suggest that newborn infants experience more pain than older infants. Early painful experiences have been shown to affect brain development and to lower pain tolerance, even years later [13]. Neonatal pain can be assessed (see Chapter 4), prevented, and treated safely using readily available nondrug and pharmacologic interventions [14].

In the first weeks of life, the way the body distributes and responds to medication is affected by several factors, including:

- Low levels of body fat and plasma proteins
- A relatively permeable blood-brain barrier
- Slow adaptive responses to hypoxia

The way the body distributes and responds to its ability to metabolize and eliminate medications is also immature, requiring lower doses and longer dosing intervals. For example, the standard pediatric dose of morphine or fentanyl is cut in half for newborns and the interval for acetaminophen is extended to every 6 or 8 hr. Whereas opioids can and should be administered when medically necessary, uncertainty about potential long-term effects reserves their use for clinical situations that cannot be managed by other means [15].

Pain Control for Routine Procedures

Healthy newborns are exposed to several routine yet painful medical procedures. Nondrug comfort measures for these procedures include:

- Sucrose pacifiers
- Topical cooling
- Massage
- Kangaroo (skin-skin contact) care
- Swaddling
- Gentle human touch

Recent, well-designed research studies have concluded that Sweet-Ease pacifiers provide relief for venipunctures but not intramuscular injections or heel lances [16]. For venipuncture, vapocoolant spray (e.g., Pain Ease) had a modest, unpredictable, but statistically significant benefit [17].

Pain Throughout Childhood

Children commonly experience acute pain due to illness, injury, and medical procedures (e.g., vaccinations). In addition to biopsychosocial aspects of pain considered for other populations, attention to developmental issues is paramount (see Table 9–1).In preverbal children, nurses rely on observational scales and surrogate reporting (usually parents) to assess for pain. Scales (e.g., the Face, Legs, Activity, Cry, Consolability [FLACC]) will not identify children who pretend to sleep as a way to cope with discomfort or fear. By ages 3 to 7, most children can reliably communicate the presence and nature of pain.

If the child is unable to communicate, behavioral indicators of pain, described in Chapter 4, in addition to the child/parent's words help guide nursing care. Even in preschool-aged children, self-report is the best method to distinguish pain from other discomforts. Use the child's own words (e.g., hurt, owie, boo-boo), and have the child point to the place that hurts. Older children can draw a picture, to aid pain-related communication.

Table 9–1 Potential Pain Amplifiers and Dampeners by Developmental Stage

AGE GROUP	POTENTIAL AMPLIFIERS	POTENTIAL DAMPENERS
Neonate	Vulnerable to cold stress Pain as a stressor Reflexive tensing to sudden stimuli Immature pain inhibiting system	Sucking reflex (sucrose pacifier) Fetal position (swaddle) Kangaroo care Music, heartbeat sounds
Infant	Muscle tension to escape pain/restraint Separation/stranger anxiety (>6 mo) Environmental extremes	Familiar voices, music Parental interaction Cuddle, rocking
Toddler and Preschooler	Fear of injury, bleeding, losing control Sadness, anxiety and/or anger Shame/guilt pain considered a punishment Cognitive distortion "magical thinking" Intense, prolonged stress Sensitization from pain earlier in life	Distraction (toys, books, pictures). Imagery ("blow away pain" with bubbles or magic, blanket/glove removes pain) Cuddling, rocking Parental interaction Reframe misconceptions, magically Listen to concerns, provide reassurance and understanding to allay fears
School-Age Child	Fear of injury, losing control/independence Sadness, anxiety and/or anger Embarassed when exposed/naked Cognitive distortion (e.g., overgeneralization) Intense, prolonged stress Regression to an earlier stage of development Sensitization from pain earlier in life	Distraction (count, tell jokes and stories, listen to music) Imagery (pleasant or guided), use volume dial (or switch) to lower pain Interaction with friends/family Reframe with rational explanations Information and behavioral rehearsal; what to expect and how it will look and feel
Adolescent	Fear of injury, losing control/independence Sadness, anxiety, and/or anger Embarassed when exposed/naked Cognitive distortion, variety of types Intense, prolonged stress; ineffective coping Sensitization from pain earlier in life	Educate about disorder/procedure and pain Provide for privacy/modesty needs Involve in decision making Distraction (music, games, TV, hobbies) Imagery (pleasant or guided), relaxation Interaction with friends > family Reframe with rational explanations

Continued

Table 9–1 Potential Pain Amplifiers and Dampeners by Developmental Stage—cont'd

AGE GROUP	POTENTIAL AMPLIFIERS	POTENTIAL DAMPENERS
Adult	Fear losing control/independence/identity Sadness, anxiety, and/or anger Cognitive distortion, variety of types Intense, prolonged stress; ineffective coping Sensitization from pain earlier in life Social isolation, role interruption/conflict Concern about what others think Fear underlying meaning of pain Spiritual distress, loss of connections	Reduce misconceptions and distortions Active involvement in control of pain Allay fears and anxiety when possible Educate about disorder/procedure and pain Involve in decision making Distraction (music, games, TV, hobbies) Imagery (pleasant or guided), relaxation Interaction with friends and family Coping skills, training Promote spiritual/meaningful connections
Elder	See adult amplifiers Declining mental capacity Heightened sensitization from unrelieved pain Multiple comorbid conditions Fatigue, insomnia/sleep disturbances Grief over multiple losses	See adult dampeners Storytelling, life review Optimize independence Altruistic endeavors

Adapted in part from unpublished information provided by Kathryn Beauchamp, RN, MS, 2008.

Treatment Modalities

Children generally respond well to multimodal therapy.

Drug Treatments

Acetaminophen is the most commonly used analgesic in children, either alone for mild pain, or combined for moderate and/or severe pain. The tolerability and safety of acetaminophen is well established; however, overdoses can damage the liver. For most children, 10 to 15 mg/kg per dose is effective, and 90 mg/kg (up to 4,000 mg) daily limit is considered safe. For newborns, a 60 mg/kg/day limit is adhered to, while preterm neonates are often limited to 45 mg/kg per day. Higher doses are used for rectal formulations because of their incomplete and variable absorption.

Ibuprofen, naproxen, and parenteral ketorolac are safe and effective in children. Aspirin is avoided in children (up to age 19) because of its association with Reye's syndrome, a potentially fatal encephalopathy. Opioid analgesics provide excellent analgesia, often with a wide safety margin, when properly dosed. Dosing is calculated using weight-based formulas (see Table 9–2), with more conservative dosing for infants under 6 months of age. Cardiopulmonary monitoring is standard when infants receive opioids [18]. Anxiolytics or sedatives are used sparingly in children as they do not relieve pain, and their side effects add safety concerns.

Nondrug Treatments

Education about what to expect and appropriate preparation for both the child and parents is helpful in controlling pain and anxiety. Quiet calm voices, lowered environmental noise and light, and confident instructions using developmentally appropriate language help maximize learning and the ability to use nondrug methods effectively.

Table 9–2	Selected Analgesic Doses Considered Safe in Opioid-Naïve Patients			
AGE	DRUG	START DOSE*	MAXIMUM/DAY	COMMENT
Neonate	Acetaminophen	10–15 mg/kg po q 8 hr	60 mg/kg Preterm 45 mg/kg	May dose q 6 hr
	Morphine	0.1 mg/kg po q 4 hr 0.03 mg/kg IV q 4 hr		
Infants and Children	Acetaminophen	10 mg/kg po q 4 hr 20 mg/kg po q 4 hr	90 mg/kg	15 mg/kg is safe May dose q 6 hr
	Ibuprofen	10 mg/kg po q 6 hr	40 mg/kg	
	Ketorolac	0.5 mg/kg IV q 6 hr	2 mg/kg	Limit to 8 doses
	Oxycodone	0.1–0.2 mg/kg q 4 hr		
	Morphine	0.3 mg/kg po q 4 hr 0.1 mg/kg IV q 4 hr		
	Hydromorphone	0.02 mg/kg IV q 1 hr		

Continued

Table 9–2 Selected Analgesic Doses Considered Safe in Opioid-Naïve Patients—cont'd

AGE	DRUG	START DOSE*	MAXIMUM/DAY	COMMENT
Adult	Acetaminophen	650 mg po q 4 hr	3,000–4,000 mg	Less with liver risk factors
	Ibuprofen	400–600 mg q 6 hr	2,400 mg	Higher dose for inflammation
	Ketorolac**	15 mg IV q 6 hr 10 mg po q 6 hr	60 mg IV 40 mg po	Limit therapy to 2–5 days
	Oxycodone	5–10 mg q 4 hr		
	Morphine	10–20 mg po q 4 hr 2–8 mg IV q 4 hr		Titrate to effect after initial dose
	Hydromorphone	2–4 mg po q 3 hr 0.5 mg IV q 3 hr		Titrate to effect after 3 doses
Older Adult	Acetaminophen	325 mg po q 4 hr or 500 mg po q 6 hr	3,000 mg/day	Less with liver risk factors
	Choline magnesium trisalicylate	500–750 mg po q 8 hr	3,000 mg/day	May decrease to once daily at steady state
	Celecoxib	100 mg BID	400 mg/day	May use cardio-protective aspirin
	Oxycodone	2.5–5 mg q 4 hr or q 6 hr		
	Morphine	2.5–10 mg po q 4 hr 1.5–5 mg IV q 4 hr		Titrate to effect after initial dose
	Hydromorphone	2 mg po q 3 hr or q 4 hr 0.5–1 mg IV q 4 hr		Titrate to effect after 3 doses

*Pediatric dosing is weight-based up to 40–60 kg, then switches to adult dosing.
**In contrast to other medications where oral doses are generally higher, the oral dose of ketorolac is lower than the IV dose due to GI toxicity.
Adapted in part from unpublished information provided by Lisa Watt, PNP, MS (2008).

Whenever possible, painful procedures should be done in a treatment room, so that the patient's room remains a safe haven. Other effective measures include:

- Using the child's security object or other distraction aids (i.e., blowing bubbles, reading pop-up books, favorite toys, and listening to music)
- Having the parent hold and talk to child, using distraction, imagery, and affirmations
- Integrating physical modalities into therapeutic play (e.g., blowing bubbles)

Cancer Pain

Cancer affects more children than any other life-limiting disease and it is more prevalent with each passing decade of life. People with cancer often experience more than one type of pain, making distinctions such as acute and chronic; or somatic, visceral, and neuropathic problematic. More than one-third of people with cancer have pain at the time of diagnosis, and 30% of cancer survivors have pain after successful treatment. In patients with advanced disease, 75% have pain. Cancer-related pain and its treatment can be prevented or satisfactorily treated in almost all cases.

The nurse should conduct a comprehensive assessment of the patient's pain, including the physical sensation and the emotional distress (see Chapter 4). Inquiring about the patient's fears, worries, sadness, or anger; and the personal and familial affects of the disease are important dimensions of pain/suffering to address. This should include:

- Patient's sources of support and strength
- Important inquiry persons or turning points in the patient's life
- Social and spiritual resources that can be mobilized during crisis

Drug Treatments

The basic approach to treating cancer pain is detailed in Chapter 6: Pharmacological Management. Pain is treated preventively or as soon as it is present, based on its intensity. Nonopioid analgesics (i.e., acetaminophen or NSAIDs) should be used, unless contraindicated. Occasionally, steroids are needed to reduce pain caused by marked inflammation or swelling. See Chapter 6 for cautions and contraindications for using NSAIDs, including risks of bleeding and masking signs of infection.

Opioids

Opioids use is indicated whenever nonopioids used alone fail to control the pain when NSAIDs are contraindicated, and/or when pain is of moderate or severe intensity. Opioids are titrated for effect using the patient's report of comfort and his or her respiratory rate as determining factors. Severe pain is treated as a medical emergency with rapid opioid titration (see Chapter 6) used to minimize the time that a pain crisis must be endured [19]. Once the pain has been controlled with short-acting opioids for more than a day, administering long-acting opioids according to a schedule controls the pain best. Short-acting opioids are then used for breakthrough pain. Further adjustments in the doses of the long-acting opioids are based on the pattern of rescue doses needed to control breakthrough pain.

Side Effects of Opioids

In some patients, the side effects of opioids (i.e., sedation, respiratory depression) are dose limiting. In those cases, multimodal therapy, regional blocks, or intrathecal analgesia are used. Although many side effects wane with ongoing therapy, constipation does not. At the start of opioid therapy, a bowel regimen is also begun. Initially a stimulant laxative and stool softener (e.g., Peri-Colace, Senokot-S) combined with diet and exercise are tried. If this is ineffective at maximum doses, a stronger stimulant laxative (bisacodyl) or an osmotic laxative (polyethylene glycol) can be tried before enemas or prokinetic agents are considered. Methylnatrexone is used if those fail to control opioids-induced constipation [20].

Adjuvant Drug Treatments

In addition to adjuvant drugs for pain control (see Chapter 4), disease or syndrome-specific treatments are used for cancer pain relief. For example, bone pain related to invasive lesions or pathological fractures is the most common cause of chronic pain with cancer. For isolated bone pain, local radiation, surgery, or nerve blocks may be used. For diffuse bone pain, chemotherapy, radiopharmaceuticals, steroids, or hormonal therapy may be used. See Box 9–2 for information on osteoblastic metastases, a common pain associated with some cancers.

Box 9–2 **Osteoblastic Metastases**

Prostate, bladder, and stomach cancers are associated with painful osteoblastic (bone-building) metastases. Radiopharmaceuticals (such as Quadramet) that slow growth and shrink tumors can relieve pain when analgesics fail. Side effects, such as bone marrow suppression or spinal compression, and toxicity limit the use of these drugs. A transient flare-up in pain during the first week often signals a therapeutic response which lessens pain for months. Urine disposal precautions are needed for 12 hr after the IV administration.

Nondrug Treatments

A variety of nondrug or complementary and alternative medicine (CAM) approaches provide symptomatic relief for persons with cancer. Many of these techniques, described in Chapter 7, are useful as adjuncts rather than replacements for medications. Additional emotional support for the patient and family is an essential part of any cancer pain treatment plan. Many organizational and community-based resources are available for cancer patients. The value of a caring nurse who takes time to sit and listen empathetically cannot be underestimated. Even when pain is difficult to control, the nurse can convey empathy and reassure the patient that the treatment team will never cease its efforts to help.

Pain in Patients With a Substance Abuse Disorder

In hospitals, 20% of all patients and 50% of those admitted with major trauma have a substance use disorder [21–23] and related pain sensitivity [24]. Addiction is a medical disorder that can be diagnosed and treated. Addiction is characterized by:

- Intense craving for the addictive substance
- Impaired control over drug use
- Compulsive use
- Continued use despite harm [25]

Clinically, patients with an active opioid addiction have a medical need for continued opioid therapy to prevent withdrawal syndrome and have rights protecting them from involuntary detoxification. Ethically, nurses have a duty to treat patients with an addiction disorder with dignity and respect, including the provision of receiving treatment for pain.

In addition to screening all patients for pain, nurses should ask every patient a drug use screening question in a nonjudgmental, respectful way. Ask about current, past, and family use of alcohol or drugs obtained without a prescription. Follow up on positive responses with focused, more detailed assessments.

There is a legitimate reluctance to start patients with an addiction disorder on opioid therapy for the management of chronic pain. NSAIDs and adjuvant drugs are considered first-line treatments for mild and moderate pain. Paradoxically, long-term opioid use may alter pain processing in a way that actually increases pain [26–28]. However, opioids are usually most effective and necessary to control severe pain regardless of drug use history.

Supervised use of opioids for treating pain will not worsen addictive disorders. Instead, failing to treat pain produces physical and emotional stress that may lead to a relapse or exacerbation of addiction [29]. Ideally, drug selection avoids the substance the patient was addicted to. The dosing schedule is designed to reduce pain and prevent the emergence of withdrawal symptoms. For some patients, it is necessary to dispense a limited number of opioids (e.g., 1-week supply) at one time.

Methadone or buprenorphine, dosed and scheduled for their analgesic effects, are good choices in this population. Advantages of methadone include:

- Low cost
- Slow development of tolerance
- Good efficacy for neuropathic pain compared with other opioids

Advantages of buprenorphine include:

- Binds more strongly to mu (μ) receptors than other opioids
- Limited euphoric and respiratory depressant effects [30]

After a dose buprenorphine, the use of unauthorized opioids or a dose escalation lowers the risk of overdose, and prevents the experience of "high" feelings.

A host of new drugs are being introduced with the hope they will prove to have abuse-deterrent properties. Added ingredients (e.g., niacin or naloxone) reduce the pleasurable effects of opioids. These drugs will likely be less desirable targets for theft or diversion for nonmedical use, however, the role of these formulas for treating pain in patients with addiction disorders is unclear.

Opioid-sparing techniques, such as adjuvant medications and nondrug techniques should be used, but not as a substitute for medically necessary analgesics. One helpful strategy is to develop a treatment plan that includes drug and nondrug techniques and have the patient self-monitor adherence to the dosing schedule and performance of functional goals. In this model, weekly continuation of opioid therapy is linked to the patient's accountability to treatment adherence and improved functioning.

Chronic Pain

Physical assessment of patients with chronic pain includes checking for:

- Allodynia
- Hyperalgesia
- Sensory, motor, and autonomic functioning
- Mental status, including cognitive and emotional functioning
- Social dysfunction and spiritual distress

Assessment of social interactions and for spiritual distress can be conducted by asking the patient open-ended questions about his or her usual and desired activities. Input from a significant other is helpful when available. Given the intractable, incurable nature of chronic pain, there is usually no single treatment that will provide more than partial, temporary relief [31]. Multimodal treatments are needed and often include:

- Adjuvant drugs, such as anticonvulsants, antidepressants, or muscle relaxants
- Analgesics, nonopioids, and/or opioids
- Nerve blocks, steroid injections, nerve lesions, and implanted devices
- Counseling

Drug Therapy

The use of long-term opioid therapy for chronic nonmalignant pain is controversial [32]. New guidelines suggest that opioids should be used as second-line therapy for treating chronic pain. In the absence of life-limiting disease, limiting daily doses to no more than 200 mg of morphine (or its equivalent) is advised. The guidelines also recommend scheduled rather than as-needed dosing. For additional breakthrough pain, nonopioid analgesics can be used on an as-needed basis [33].

Multidisciplinary Approaches

To offset the risk of disability and depression, multidisciplinary rehabilitation may offer the best hope for optimizing functioning. Active self-management techniques must be part of any chronic pain treatment plan, so the patient has access to a variety of self-initiated skills (i.e., pacing activities or self-hypnosis) to help control the pain when needed. Multiple interventions must be used concurrently to address the needs of the body, mind, spirit, and social interactions (see Chapter 8). Adaptive equipment also may be needed to optimize independence and functioning.

Wellness behaviors can be integrated into the treatment plan to help reverse some of the secondary problems commonly resulting from changes in diet, exercise, stress, and sleep [34, 35]. Therapies that minimize the negative effect of stress, disabling beliefs, and upsetting emotions must be mastered over time with multiple education and counseling sessions. Cognitive-behavioral treatment (CBT) programs provide the structure, guidance, and reinforcement necessary for long-term success [36, 37].

Interventions directed at the spiritual domain are an outgrowth of the spiritual assessment. For those who express their spirituality in a religious context, offering prayer or access to meaningful rituals is appropriate [38].

For others, caring presence, attentive listening, and facilitating the process of acceptance can help reduce spiritual distress [39, 40]. Many patients with chronic pain harbor unresolved grief. Grieving helps patients form a new identity and set realistic goals that strive to restore joy, function, and meaning.

Pain in the Older Adult

Aging alters many physiologic processes, resulting in increased pain thresholds, increased sensitization, and weakened responses in descending inhibitory circuits [41]. This impairs the ability to recover from hyperalgesic or allodynic states [41, 42] while increasing the risk of chronic pain. Ironically, some changes that occur with advancing age fail to send needed pain signals to alert the older adult of a heart attack or GI obstruction [43–45]. For example, nearly two-thirds of older adults report an absence of pain or an atypical presentation during a heart attack [46].

Because of these vulnerabilities, nurses should screen every elderly patient for discomfort. The Numeric Rating Scale, Verbal Descriptor Scale, and Faces Pain Scale (revised) are the best established tools for alert, cognitively intact older adults. The Iowa Pain Thermometer demonstrated comparable results and was preferred by older adults [47, 48]. Tips for using all these scales include:

- Substitute the word "discomfort" for "pain"
- Overcome sensory deficits (eyeglasses, hearing aids, large font/bold print)
- Determine if the patient understands the scale before using it

Drug Therapy

The older adult's body composition (less water and more fat than in younger adults) favors the distribution and accumulation of fat-soluble drugs, such as fentanyl. Lower-serum protein levels increase the bioavailability of highly protein-bound drugs (e.g., aspirin or ibuprofen), especially in patients who take multiple drugs. The liver and kidneys are smaller and have reduced capacity to metabolize and eliminate drugs, which limits the production of active metabolites and prolongs the duration of action, while raising the risk of side effects and toxicity [49].

Acetaminophen is the first-line analgesic of choice for older patients [52] with mild or moderate pain. It may be less effective than other nonopioids, but it is considered safer in all patients EXCEPT in those who:

- Are taking warfarin
- Have impaired renal function

- Are dehydrated
- Suffer from chronic alcoholism or have liver disease

Dosage limits of 2 to 3 g per day will minimize risk of toxicity. Because acetaminophen is in many other drugs, care must be taken to avoid inadvertent exposure. Adding or substituting an occasional NSAID will provide superior analgesia. Limits on the dose and duration of NSAID therapy (lowest effective dose for no more than 10 days) are advised to prevent significant bleeding, GI, cardiovascular, and renal problems.

Opioid therapy is safe and effective for older adults for moderate and severe pain. Starting doses are 50% to 75% lower than in younger adults, and intervals between doses are longer, especially in patients with renal or hepatic disease [53]. Respiratory depression occurs infrequently, unless doses are too high or are increased too rapidly. At greatest risk are patients with preexisting respiratory, renal, or kidney dysfunction and those with untreated sleep apnea. Opioids also can cause peripheral vasodilatation, leading to orthostatic hypotension and thus increasing the risk of falling.

ALERT

The Beers criteria, developed to raise awareness of medications that should not be used by older adults, identifies all NSAIDs, nonselective and COX-2 selective, as drugs to avoid. Indomethacin—and ketorolac in particular—carry the greatest risk of life-threatening GI bleeding. Opioids as a class did not make the list, but propoxyphene, meperidine, and pentazocine are listed to be avoided in the elderly because of neurological and cardiovascular toxicity [50, 51].

Despite those risks, long-term use of opioids poses a lower risk of life-threatening events than sustained NSAID therapy [52]. Excluding constipation, other common side effects, diminish over the first couple of weeks of therapy. Many elders worry that opioids will cloud their thinking, but uncontrolled pain is 9 times more likely to produce delirium in older adults than are opioids [54].

Oxycodone, hydromorphone, and morphine are probably the best first-line analgesics for opioid-naïve older patients with acute pain. Starting doses are 2.5 mg of oxycodone, 5 mg of oral morphine, or 1 to 2 mg of parenteral morphine. Although morphine can be titrated more quickly, generally the short-acting opioids are titrated on a daily basis, while long-acting products can be safely titrated once or twice a week [55]. In Europe, buprenorphine is emerging as a potential first-line opioid with desirable pharmacokinetic and pharmacodynamic properties in older adults. The absorption, distribution, metabolism, and excretion of buprenorphine, and the ceiling to its respiratory depressant effects make it a good choice for older adults [30]. The lack of oral formulations for pain in the U.S. limits its use.

Age-Appropriate Therapeutic Selections: Drugs to Avoid

Propoxyphene, meperidine, and pentazocine are drugs to avoid in the elderly because they are neurotoxic, resulting in confusion, agitation, and possible seizures. Propoxyphene is as weak as aspirin but has cardiotoxic and neurotoxic effects [51]. Meperidine analgesia is brief, but its toxic metabolite (normeperidine) remains for days. At doses of 600 mg per day, or if used for more than 48 hr it causes seizures in most elders.

To promote safe, effective pain control in older adults, consider the following choices:

- Use gabapentin or pregabalin as first-line for neuropathic pain
- If antidepressants are needed, use duloxetine or desipramine, not amitriptyline
- Consider trying topical drugs (diclofenac, lidocaine, or capsaicin) for localized pain
- Therapeutic exercise and aquatic therapy are preferred over topical heat or transcutaneous electrical nerve stimulation (TENS) [41, 56]

Nondrug Therapies

Many older persons embrace CAM, especially prayer/energy medicine and the use of herbs or biological therapies. As with younger patients, multidisciplinary, multimodal approaches to pain relief have better outcomes than treatment approaches that rely on only single modalities [57, 58].

Pain at the End of Life

Pain at the end of life typically is present in combination with other discomforts. Concurrent social isolation, spiritual distress, family anxiety, grief, and decisions regarding the use of life-extending technologies add to the complexity. Nurses working with these patients and families need to expand their assessment of pain to include physical, cognitive, emotional, social, and spiritual dimensions. When the patient can no longer verbalize his or her experience, nurses use a combination of behavioral observation, surrogate reporting, and knowledge of the patient's condition to anticipate and meet comfort needs.

Although pain is the most common distressing symptom at the end of life, patients also commonly experience:

- Fatigue
- Anorexia

- Nausea
- Weakness
- Dyspnea
- Altered mental status
- Abnormal bowel and bladder function

Many pain medications can cause or worsen these symptoms, and patients often refuse pain medications when they believe analgesics make other symptoms worse.

In an ideal situation, symptom clusters can be managed with one medication that treats more than one symptom. For example, morphine can be titrated to best reduce pain, cough, and dyspnea. Sometimes, switching drugs can improve symptom clusters, such as choosing transdermal fentanyl instead of a long-acting oral opioid for constipated patients. In other circumstances, using adjuvant drugs to manage side effects may secondarily reduce opioid requirements. In the uncommon situation where pain cannot be relieved without worsening other symptoms, regional or spinal interventions are a viable option. When pain and agitation persist, palliative sedation may be considered.

As the end of life nears, multiple organ system failures often develop. When the kidneys begin to fail, morphine or other opioids with potentially toxic metabolites should be switched to those without that problem. NSAIDs also must be stopped, because they further damage kidneys, and hasten the process of renal failure. When the GI system fails, oral medications are switched to other routes. When the liver begins to fail, analgesic dosing intervals are increased and doses are lowered carefully to maintain analgesia level, while minimizing the risk of side effects or toxicity.

At the end of life, caregiver support is an important part of care. Nurses should teach caregivers about the medication regimen and about nondrug comfort measures. Caregivers often experience high levels of physical and emotional stress as their loved one approaches death. Often they remain at the dying person's side at the expense of their own needs or those of other family members. Nurses often arrange for home support services and respite care whenever these services are available.

ALERT

With renal impairment, avoid NSAIDs because they reduce renal circulation and damage glomeruli. Opioids with active (codeine) or toxic (meperidine, propoxyphene) metabolites also are avoided to prevent their accumulation. With liver disease, acetaminophen is avoided because it advances hepatic damage, and drugs with active metabolites are avoided because the liver cannot process them. Fentanyl may be best in both cases because it lacks active or toxic metabolites, and is excreted in the stool.

In conclusion, nurses have a duty to recognize and relieve pain in patients they serve, regardless of age, stage of life, or diagnosis. Through direct patient care, coordinating services with other professionals, and advocacy; nurses can improve the care of patients with uncontrolled pain right now. As Dr. Ira Byok, Professor and Director of Palliative Care at Dartmouth Medical School asks, "If not now, when? If not here, where?" "If not us, who will do this important work?" (personal communication, October 18, 2006). As nurses, we are well positioned to ensure that high-quality care is provided to all patients, wherever and whenever they report pain.

10 Tools

Dos and Don'ts of Pain
Management   page 217

Sample Assessment Questions:
Acute Pain Using WILDA Acronym   page 218

Suggested Starting Doses
of First-Line Analgesics
for Opioid-Naïve Adult Patients   page 219

Equianalgesic Chart   page 220

Determining Starting Doses
When Switching Opioids   page 221

Fentanyl Transdermal (TD) Patch
Equianalgesic Conversion   page 222

Spectrum of Pain Relief Options   page 223

Nondrug Pain Relief/Comforting
Checklist   page 224

Nondrug Sleep Hygiene with Pain   page 225

Considerations When Refining
an Ineffective Pain Treatment Plan   page 226

Pain Management Flow Sheet   page 228

Pain Assessment/Reassessment
Chart Audit   page 230

Resources for Advancing Safe,
Effective Pain Control   page 231

Tools

Tools

Dos and Don'ts of Pain Management

The following six "Do" instructions will help to improve patient comfort and satisfaction, while avoiding six "Don't" pitfalls will minimize treatment failures and conflict.

Do

- Ask the patient about pain and use valid assessment tools appropriate for the patient
- Accept the patient's report of pain as the best available indication of need
- Use treatments likely to be effective for the type and intensity of pain
- Offer prn medications on a schedule for patients with severe/persistent pain
- Use adjuvant medications, nonopioids, and nondrug methods to supplement opioids
- Anticipate, monitor for, and treat analgesic side effects

Don't

- Don't expect all patients to have the same analgesic requirements
- Don't establish a pain treatment plan without involving the patient
- Don't use codeine, meperidine, propoxyphene, or the IM route when better options are available
- Don't label patients as "drug-seeking" based solely on their request for pain relief
- Don't perpetuate common fears and misconceptions about opioids
- Don't work alone

Sample Assessment Questions: Acute Pain Using WILDA Acronym

After screening the patient and getting an affirmative response to the question, "Are you having any discomfort right now?" Ask the following additional questions:

Words (description of the discomfort, such as sharp or aching)
- What word best describes your discomfort?

Intensity (severity of pain)
- How strong (intense) is your pain? (use *one* of the scales below)
  - On a scale of 0–10, with 0 as no pain and 10 as the worst imaginable
  - Is it mild, moderate, severe, or extreme
    - Clinician rates as 2, 4, 6, and 8 respectively
    - Note: 0 = no pain and 10 = worst imaginable, as above
  - To what extent does it interfere with your activities?
    - No interference (2)
    - Interferes with some activities (4)
    - Interferes with all actions requiring exertion (6)
    - Interferes with even passive actions, such as talking or reading (8)
    - Cannot even speak, in too much pain (10)

Location (body parts that are uncomfortable)
- Where specifically are you feeling the discomfort?

Duration (pattern of pain over time)
- When did the discomfort start?
- How has it changed over time?
- Is it constant or intermittent?
- Is your discomfort better or worse at specific times of the day?

Aggravating and Alleviating factors
- What makes the discomfort worse?
- What makes you feel better? (e.g., medication, specific movements, or activities, etc.)

Suggested Starting Doses of First-Line Analgesics for Opioid-Naïve Adult Patients*

MEDICATION	ORAL	PARENTERAL	DOSE INTERVAL	MAXIMUM SAFE DOSE
NONOPIOIDS (MILD PAIN)				
Acetaminophen (APAP)	500–650 mg		q 4 or q 6 hr	Limit APAP to 2,000–4,000 mg/day**
Ibuprofen	200–400 mg		q 6 hr	2,400 mg/day
Naproxen Sodium	550 mg start, then 250 mg		q 8 hr	1,650 mg/day
COMBINATION OPIOID-NONOPIOIDS (MODERATE PAIN)				
Codeine	30–60 mg	N/A	q 3 or q 4 hr	Limit codeine to 60 mg/dose Limit APAP to 2–4 g/day**
Hydrocodone (e.g., Lorcet, Lortab, Vicodin)	5–10 mg	N/A	q 3 or q 4 hr	Limit APAP to 2–4 g/day**
Oxycodone (e.g., Roxicodone, Percocet, Tylox, Norco)	5 mg	N/A	q 3 or q 4 hr	Limit APAP to 2–4 g/day**
OPIOID AGONIST (MODERATE TO SEVERE PAIN)				
Morphine	10–30 mg	2–10 mg	q 3 or q 4 hr	Individual, adjust doses by 25%–50% at a time, never increasing by more than twofold at one time
Hydromorphone (Dilaudid)	2–7.5 mg	0.5–1.5 mg	q 3 or q 4 hr	Same as morphine
Oxycodone	5–20 mg	N/A	q 3 or q 4 hr	Same as morphine

*Starting doses for older adults are 50% lower than those displayed. Weight-based dosing is used for children.
**APAP limit is 4 g per day for otherwise young healthy patients. The 2-g per day limit is for dehydrated, hepatic disease, or alcoholism.
Data from American Pain Society (APS). (2008). *Principles of analgesic use in the treatment of acute pain and cancer pain, 6th ed.* Glenview, IL: APS Press.

Equianalgesic Chart

DRUG	PARENTERAL DOSE	ORAL DOSE	COMMENTS
Morphine	10 mg	30 mg	Higher oral doses may be needed early in therapy (1:6, IV:oral ratio)
Meperidine	75 mg	300 mg	Avoid multiple-dose use due to toxic effects
Fentanyl	0.1 mg (100 mcg)	100 mcg (buccal)	Standard starting dose (100 mcg buccal) only for breakthrough pain in opioid-tolerant patients
Dilaudid (HYDRO-morPHONE)	1.5 mg	7.5 mg	The brand name and special TALLman lettering is used because hydromorphone is the most common drug cited in sound-alike, look-alike (wrong drug) errors.
Hydrocodone	N/A	20 mg	Nonopioid ingredient limits dose
Codeine	130 mg	200 mg	Doses listed are higher than the analgesic ceiling and maximum tolerated dose of 60 mg for most patients
Oxymorphone	1 mg	10 mg	This drug may be more potent in older adults or when taken with food or alcohol
Oxycodone	N/A	20 mg	Available in combination products and as a single agent (both immediate release or sustained release), enhancing its utility

$$\frac{\text{Equianalgesic Table dose of current drug}}{\text{Equianalgesic Table dose of new drug}} = \frac{24° \text{ dose current drug}}{X\ (24° \text{ dose new drug})}$$

Determining Starting Doses When Switching Opioids

Step 1: Determine the total current 24-hour opioid requirement based on use in past 24–48 hours:

(NOTE: If more than one agent used, need to convert each drug to a morphine equivalent.)

Total opioid needed/day = _____ day.

Step 2: Set up an equianalgesic equation:

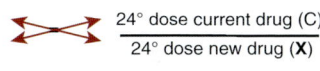

$$\frac{\text{Equianalgesic Table dose of current drug}}{\text{Equianalgesic Table dose of new drug}} \left(\frac{A}{B}\right) = \frac{24° \text{ dose current drug}}{24° \text{ dose new drug}} \left(\frac{C}{X}\right)$$

Step 3: Solve for **X**:

$$\frac{\text{Equianalgesic Table dose of current drug (A)}}{\text{Equianalgesic Table dose of new drug (B)}} \diagdown\diagup \frac{24° \text{ dose current drug (C)}}{24° \text{ dose new drug (X)}}$$

a) A**X** = BC
b) **X** = BC/A
c) **X** = 24 hour anticipated need of new drug in mg (or mcg)

Step 4: Decrease by 25%–50% for incomplete cross-tolerance **unless**:
   Switching route not drug
   Patient has severe unrelieved pain
   Patient has not been on medication long enough to develop tolerance
   Fentanyl or methadone is being used (different calculation method)

Step 5: Consider how new medication is supplied to determine starting dose and schedule

Step 6: Add prn rescue dosing 10%–20% daily dose available q2h

Thus the calculated safe, effective starting point based on how the medication is supplied:

Step 7: Monitor patient closely for balance of analgesia, function, and side effects

Step 8: In 24 hours review total dose received, effect, and recalculate scheduled dose as indicated

Fentanyl Transdermal (TD) Patch Equianalgesic Conversion*

TRANSDERMAL FENTANYL (MCG/HR)	PARENTERAL MORPHINE EQUIVALENT (MG/HR) TO TD FENTANYL	ORAL MORPHINE EQUIVALENT (MG/DAY) TO TD FENTANYL	PARENTERAL (DILAUDID) EQUIVALENT (MG/HR) TO TD FENTANYL	ORAL OXYCODONE EQUIVALENT (MG/DAY) TO TD FENTANYL	MANUFACTURER'S RANGE FOR ORAL MORPHINE EQUIVALENT (MG/DAY) TO TD FENTANYL	APS GUIDE TO POTENCY CONVERSIONS FROM ORAL MORPHINE (MG/DAY) TO TD FENTANYL
12** mcg/hr	0.3 mg/hr	45 mg/day	0.05 mg/hr	20 mg/day		
25** mcg/hr	0.6 mg/hr	90 mg/day	0.1 mg/hr	45 mg/day	60–134 mg/day	30–90 mg/day
50** mcg/hr	1.3 mg/hr	180 mg/day	0.2 mg/hr	90 mg/day	135–224 mg/day	91–150 mg/day
75** mcg/hr	1.8 mg/hr	270 mg/day	0.3 mg/hr	135 mg/day	225–314 mg/day	151–210 mg/day
100** mcg/hr	2.5 mg/hr	360 mg/day	0.4 mg/hr	180 mg/day	315–404 mg/day	211–270 mg/day
125 mcg/hr	3.1 mg/hr	450 mg/day	0.5 mg/hr	225 mg/day	405–494 mg/day	271–330 mg/day
150 mcg/hr	3.7 mg/hr	540 mg/day	0.6 mg/hr	270 mg/day	495–584 mg/day	331–390 mg/day
175 mcg/hr	4.3 mg/hr	630 mg/day	0.7 mg/hr	315 mg/day	585–674 mg/day	391–450 mg/day
200 mcg/hr	5 mg/hr	720 mg/day	0.8 mg/hr	360 mg/day	675–764 mg/day	451–510 mg/day
225 mcg/hr	5.5 mg/hr	810 mg/day	0.8 mg/hr	400 mg/day	765–854 mg/day	511–570 mg/day
250 mcg/hr	6.3 mg/hr	900 mg/day	0.9 mg/hr	450 mg/day	855–944 mg/day	571–630 mg/day
275 mcg/hr	6.8 mg/hr	990 mg/day	1 mg/hr	500 mg/day	945–1,034 mg/day	631–690 mg/day
300 mcg/hr	7.4 mg/hr	1080 mg/day	1.1 mg/hr	540 mg/day	1,035–1,124 mg/day	691–750 mg/day

*Note: Doses listed here are approximately at the midpoint of the range provided by the manufacturer.
The manufacturer bases the conversion to TD Fentanyl on conservative estimates compared with those of the American Pain Society (APS) analgesic guidelines (2008).
** 12 mcg/hr patch delivers 12.5 mcg/hr, however "12 label" minimizes "wrong dose" (125 mcg/hr) errors.

Spectrum of Pain Relief Options*

SELF-INITIATED OR "LOW-TECH" APPROACHES	TREATMENT TARGETS (AND COMMON MEDICATIONS)	PROFESSIONAL–INITIATED OR "HIGH-TECH" APPROACHES
IMMEDIATE AREA OF PAIN		
Massage, rubbing Moist heat Application ice Positioning Braces, orthotics, compression Remove source, cause of pain	Medications: 　NSAIDs 　Cause-directed 　Capsaicin or menthol 　cream	Physical therapy (modalities) Electric stimulation (TENS) Specialized massage techniques Trigger point injections Laser therapy Surgery
REGION OF PAIN OR SPINE		
Reduce dermatonal stimuli Contralateral stimulation Proximal/distal stimulation	Medications: 　Opioids 　Anticonvulsants 　Antidepressants 　Other coanalgesics	Nerve blocks (sensory, autonomic) Cryotherapy, radiofrequency Prolotherapy (sugar injected in tendons) Peripheral nerve stimulation Spinal cord stimulation Epidural/spinal analgesia Physical manipulation, traction
WHOLE BODY		
Diet, nutritional supplements Exercise, pacing activities Herbal or aroma therapy Breathing techniques		Acupuncture, acupressure Work hardening Functional restoration Multidisciplinary rehabilitation
BRAIN OR MIND-BODY FOCUSED		
Relaxation, imagery, hypnosis Knowledge about condition Music, distraction Journal writing Change thinking, attitudes Reduce fear, anxiety, stress Reduce sadness, helplessness	Medications: 　Opioids 　Anticonvulsants 　Antidepressants 　Other coanalgesics	Biofeedback training Counseling Electroconvulsive therapy Deep-brain stimulation Cognitive-behavioral therapy

Continued

Spectrum of Pain Relief Options*—cont'd

SELF-INITIATED OR "LOW-TECH" APPROACHES	TREATMENT TARGETS (AND COMMON MEDICATIONS)	PROFESSIONAL–INITIATED OR "HIGH-TECH" APPROACHES
SPIRITUAL OR ENERGY-FOCUSED		
Prayer, meditation Self-reflection, re: life/pain Meaningful rituals Energy work (e.g., TT, reiki)		Spiritual healing Magnetic therapy Homeopathic remedies
SOCIAL INTERACTION-FOCUSED		
Improved communication Volunteering Problem solving Support groups Pet therapy		Family therapy Functional restoration Vocational training Psychosocial counseling

*Organized by target of action and level of invasiveness

Nondrug Pain Relief/Comforting Checklist

KNOW CAN USE	LIKE TO KNOW	LIKE TO TRY LEARN	TREATMENT APPROACH
			Area of Pain—Skin Level
			Reducing pain triggers
			Massage, chiropractic care
			Applying heat or cold to pain
			Electric stimulation (TENS)
			Positioning, brace, orthotics
			Acupuncture, acupressure
			Spinal Level
			Reduce local nerve irritation
			Good posture and alignment
			Skin stimulation–not on pain (proximal, distal, contralateral)
			Whole Body Level
			Diet, nutritional supplements
			Exercise, pacing activities
			Adequate sleep, rest
			Fresh air, clean water

Nondrug Pain Relief/Comforting Checklist—cont'd

KNOW CAN USE	LIKE TO KNOW	LIKE TO TRY LEARN	TREATMENT APPROACH
			Mind Level
			Relaxation, imagery
			Information about pain
			Pain diary, journal writing
			Distracting attention (music, humor, reading, hobbies)
			Rethinking situation
			Attitude adjustment
			Reduce fear, anxiety, stress
			Reduce sadness, helplessness
			Social and/or Spiritual Level
			Prayer, meditation
			Reminiscence
			Meaningful rituals
			Energy work (e.g., TT, rekki)
			Spiritual healing
			Restoration relationships
			Improved communication
			Family activities
			Presence of caring person
			Volunteering
			Support groups

Nondrug Sleep Hygiene with Pain*

IN COMMUNITY	IN HOSPITAL
Consistent wake time	Limit early morning light/noise
Bright light in the morning for 30 min	Bright light in the morning for 30 min
Use bed only for sleep and sexual activity	Avoid doing painful procedures in bed
Limit daytime napping to 20–30 min	Limit daytime nap duration to 90 min
Exercise 30–40 min per day	Daytime activity appropriate to condition
Avoid evening caffeine, alcohol, nicotine	Avoid evening caffeine, alcohol, nicotine

Nondrug Sleep Hygiene with Pain*—cont'd

IN COMMUNITY	IN HOSPITAL
Avoid large, spicy, or fatty snacks	Avoid large, spicy, or fatty evening snacks
Bath 1–2 hr before bedtime	PM care with back rub if desired
Adjust temperature for cooling trend	Limit ambient light and noise as possible
Allow 30–60 min for bedtime routine	Night routine that limits interruptions
Reduce exposure to noise and lights	Read or listen to relaxing music, not TV if awake
Turn clock away or remove from bedside	Promote physical/emotional comfort
If awake** read or listen to relaxing music, not TV	

*Time pain medications in a way that promotes relief during normal sleep time.
**If awake more than 30 min, redose analgesic if appropriate and change activity for 30 min then reattempt sleeping.

Considerations When Refining an Ineffective Pain Treatment Plan

Step 1: Review assessments and treatment plans to determine if further analysis is needed
- Have new or different diagnoses emerged?
- Is the patient's goal for comfort and functioning realistic?
- What barriers to pain relief have been identified? Which have been addressed?
- What emotional distresses have been identified? Which have been addressed?

Step 2: Analyze the alignment of the treatment with the pain type
- Are NSAIDs being used for mild pain or aches or as part of multimodal therapy?
- Are mixed/weak opioids being used for moderate pain?
- Are strong opioids being used for severe pain?
- Are adjuvants directed at the cause or for calming pain-generating nerves?

- Have medications been administered consistently enough to achieve a steady state?

Step 3: Consider the merit of changing the regimen, discuss with pharmacist and prescriber
- If ineffective or not tolerated, has switching the drug been considered?
- If a dose-response relationship was noted, has a dosage adjustment been tried?
- If effective intermittently have adjustments using the same drug been tried such as:
  - Scheduling ATC rather than PRN dosing?
  - Long-acting agent for constant pain with a known effective dose?

Step 4: Implement the refined analgesic regimen
- Are analgesics consistently offered on schedule?
- Are there 2 or more consecutive pain score ratings below the pain scale midpoint?
- Does dose adjustment $+/- 25\%-50\%$ achieve acceptable levels of comfort/side effects?
  - Work within limits of range order or secure revised order
- Add coanalgesics/adjuvants as ordered to target multiple mechanisms and cut side effects
- Document interventions and timely evaluations of responses to guide further refinement

Step 5: Use nondrug techniques to compliment the analgesic regimen
- Have a variety of techniques been tried?
- Has the technique the patient believes to be most effective been tried?
- Does reducing emotional distress also reduce pain levels?

Step 6: Access available resources (e.g., pain specialists) and referrals for advanced techniques

Pain Management Flow Sheet

Sample developed to document multiple analgesic orders or technologies with monitoring guidance

ID# for ordering	Allergy:		Analgesic Ordered:	Drug(s):	Dose:	Route:	Interval:
			Monitoring Required:	Elements in instruction box below on left:		Also monitor:	
ORDER		Date					
MONITORING		Time					
		Respiratory Rate					
		O₂ Sat					
		Pain Score (0-10)					
		Sedation Score (S-4)					
		Sensory Score (0-2)					
		Motor Score (0-5)					
		Side Effects (N,V,R,I,T,C)					
		Order verified by second RN					
INTRAVENOUS		Drug					
		Basal (continuous) Rate					
		Bolus (mg)					
		Lockout					
		1 hour limit					
		Shift Total Volume (ml)					
		Shift Total Dose (mg)					

PAIN SCORE:
0 ——— 10
NO PAIN   WORST PAIN IMAGINABLE

See pain guidelines for numeric & behavioral scales

SIDE EFFECTS:
N = Nausea   I = Itching
V = Vomiting   T = Tinnitus
R = Urinary Retention   C = Confused

SENSORY SCORE:
Indicate R=right; L=left, or B=Bilateral
0 = No numbness, no decreased sensation
1 = No numbness with decreased sensation
2 = Numbness and decreased or no sensation

MOTOR SCORE:
Indicate R=right; L=left, or B=Bilateral
0 = No movement – no contraction
1 = Muscle flicker but no movement
2 = Moves on bed (horizontal), not against gravity
3 = Moves against gravity, not resistance
4 = Moves against some examiner resistance
5 = Normal strength

Continued

SEDATION SCORE:
S = Sleeping, easy to arouse
1 = Alert & awake
2 = Slightly drowsy
3 = Drowsy, arouses briefly, nods off
4 = Somnolent, difficult to arouse

INSTRUCTIONS:
1. Pain, Sedation & Respiratory Rate q1h x 4h, then q4h until catheter is discontinued (DC'd).
2. Sensory & Motor Score q1h x 4h, then q2h until spinal/peripheral nerve catheter DC'd.
3. Total the dose q8h or when new syringe is hung.
4. Order verification when new bag is hung.
5. If order is changed/discontinued note clearly.

SEEK ASSISTANCE FOR:
- Pain score greater than 6 (0-10 scale)
- New onset pain at insertion site (e.g. back pain).
- RR less than 10.
- Sedation Score of 3 or 4.
- New or progressive sensory/motor deficits.
- Side effects unrelieved by ordered drugs.
- BP 50 mm Hg below systolic baseline.
- Temperature >101°F (38.5°C).
- Dressing saturated or catheter displaced.

Other route (please circle)															
Epidural Intrathecal Peripheral Nerve															
Drug															
Catheter Site															
Basal (Continuous) Rate															
Bolus															
Lockout															
1 hour limit															
Shift Total Volume (ml)															
Shift Total Dose (mg)															
ROUTINE Drug															
PRNS Drug															
BOLUSES Drug															
Other Therapy:															
Other Therapy:															
Initials:															

INITIALS	FULL SIGNATURE	INITIALS	FULL SIGNATURE	INITIALS	FULL SIGNATURE

Pain Assessment/Reassessment Chart Audit

Date_____ Unit _____ Room # _____ MRN _____ Auditor _____

# Required	# Performed	Indicator	Criteria
On admission and 1/transfer		Pain is assessed on admission	Check admission record for pain assessment on arrival to facility/unit
1/shift		Pain assessment each shift	Over a 24-hour period: How many pain assessments are documented?
# of interventions		Pain relief interventions recorded **Pain Meds Administered** Times:	Look at progress notes and medication records Count # of interventions, & time of meds
1 reassessment for each intervention		Reassessment Entries (analgesic effect/side effect)	Look at flowsheet and progress notes for an entry after each pain-relief intervention

Patients with clinically significant pain (rated >5/10):

Was it resolved (2 consecutive reading <5) ever? ____yes ____no

Was it resolved (2 consecutive reading <5) within 24h? ____yes ____no

Were opioids used? (morphine, oxycodone, dilaudid, fentanyl) ____yes ____no

Were non-opioid drugs used? (aspirin, tylenol, toradol) ____yes ____no

Were adjuvant drugs used? (neurontin, lidoderm, elavil) ____yes ____no

Were nondrug methods used? ____yes ____no
(circle: Heat/cold, massage, distraction, positioning, relaxation, other)

Was the treatment plan revised? ____yes ____no

Comments or Follow-up:

RESOURCES FOR ADVANCING SAFE, EFFECTIVE PAIN CONTROL

The art, science, and standards of professional practice pertaining to pain are advancing at a rapid pace. Those committed to providing optimal pain relief also are dedicated to lifelong learning. New resources are constantly emerging, so the prudent clinician is urged to keep abreast of latest developments in the field. The following resources were selected as the most helpful and current at the time of publication. Additional resources are included to help the nurse find updated content as it becomes available. Given the plethora of information available and the desire to not confuse or overwhelm the reader, each type of resource is limited to no more than a dozen options.

SELECTED CLINICAL PRACTICE GUIDELINES

Miaskowski, C., Cleary J., Burney, R., Coyne, P., Finley, R., Foster, R., et al. (2005). *Guideline for the management of cancer pain in adults and children,* APS Clinical Practice Guideline Series, No 3. Glenview, IL: American Pain Society.

Hadjistavropoulos, T., Herr, K., Turk, D.C., et al. (2007). An interdisciplinary expert consensus statement on assessment of pain in older persons. *Clinical Journal of Pain,* 23(1):S1–S43.

American Geriatrics Society. AGS Panel on the Pharmacological Management of Persistent Pain in Older Persons. (2009) Pharmacological Management of Persistent Pain in Older Persons. *J Am Geriatr Soc.* 2009 Aug, 57:1331–1346.

Simon, L.S., Lipman, A.G., Jacox, A, et al. (2002). *Guideline for the management of pain in osteoarthritis, rheumatoid arthritis, and juvenile chronic arthritis* (2nd ed.). Glenview, IL: American Pain Society.

American Society of Anesthesiologists Task Force on Acute Pain Management (2004).

Practice guidelines for acute pain management in the perioperative setting. *Anesthesiology,* 100:1573–1581.

National Comprehensive Cancer Network. (2007). Pediatric cancer pain. Retrieved January 7, 2009 from http://www.nccn.org/professionals/physician_gls/ PDF/pediatric_pain.pdf Adult (2008) version http://www.nccn.org/professionals/ physician_gls/PDF/pain.pdf

Dworkin, R.H., O'Connor, A.B., Backonja, M., et al. (2007). Pharmacologic management of neuropathic pain: Evidence-based recommendations. Pain, (Dec 5);132(3):237–251. Retrieved August 26, 2009 from http://www.guideline. gov/summary/pdf.aspx?doc_id=11724&stat=1&string=

Burckhardt, C.S., Goldenberg, D., Crofford, L., et al. (2005). *Guideline for the management of fibromyalgia syndrome pain in adults and children.* Glenview, IL: American Pain Society.

Chou, R., Qaseem, A., Snow, V., Casey, D., Cross, T., Shekelle, P., et al. (2007). Diagnosis and treatment of low back pain: A joint clinical practice guideline from the American College of Physicians and the American Pain Society. *Annals of Internal Medicine, 147*(7): 478–491.

Chou, R., & Huffman, L.H. (2007). Nonpharmacologic therapies for acute and chronic low back pain: A review of the evidence for an American Pain Society/American College of Physicians clinical practice guideline. *Annals of Internal Medicine*, 147(7):492–504.

Chou, R., Loeser, J.D., Owens, D.K. (for the American Pain Society Guidelines Panel). (2009). Interventional therapies, surgery, and interdisciplinary rehabilitation for low back pain: An evidence-based clinical practice guideline from the American Pain Society. *Spine, 34*(10):1066–1077.

Chou, R., Fanciullo, G.J., Fine, P.G., et al. (2009). Clinical guidelines for the use of chronic opioid therapy in chronic noncancer pain: American Pain Society & American Academy of Pain Medicine opioids guidelines panel. *Journal of Pain, 10*:113–146.

Shaiova, L., Berger, A., Blinderman, C.D., et al. (2008). Consensus guideline on parenteral methadone use in pain and palliative care. *Palliative and Supportive Care, 6*:165–176.

PAIN ORGANIZATIONS OF INTEREST TO PROFESSIONAL NURSES

American Society for Pain Management Nursing—an organization dedicated to advance and promote optimal nursing care for people affected by pain through education, standards, advocacy, and research. Certification programs, practice guidelines, position papers and local chapters are available. P.O. Box 15473, Lenexa, KS 66285–5473 http://www.aspmn.org/

American Pain Society—a multidisciplinary pain organization advancing research, education, treatment, and professional practice for pain in general and special interest groups (e.g., pediatric, nursing, forensics, etc.). Local chapters are listed on Web site. 4700 W. Lake Avenue, Glenview, IL 60025 http://www.ampainsoc.org/

International Association for the Study of Pain (IASP)—unites scientists, clinicians, and policy makers from around the world. It stimulates research conduct and utilization, funds international collaborative projects, and holds a World Congress on even years. 111 Queen Anne Avenue N., Suite 501, Seattle, WA 98109–4955 http://www.iasp-pain.org/

Alliance of State Pain Initiatives—national organization that promotes pain relief nationwide by supporting the efforts of state and regional pain initiatives. 1300 University Avenue, Room 4720, Madison, WI 53706 http://www.aacpi.org/

American Academy of Pain Management—a national multidisciplinary pain society that provide credentialing to practitioners regardless of discipline. Mission is to serve those who treat people with pain through education, setting standards of care, and advocacy. 13947 Mono Way #A, Sonora, CA 95370 http://www.aapainmanage.org/

Hospice and Palliative Nurses Association (HPNA)—professional nursing organization dedicated to promoting excellence in hospice and palliative nursing care. Excellent resources, links to educators, position papers, and mentoring opportunities. One Penn Center West, Suite 229, Pittsburgh, PA 152706–0100 http://www.hpna.org

Oncology Nursing Society—a professional nursing organization dedicated to excellence in patient care, education, research, and administration in oncology nursing. Many useful resources including the evidence-based "PEP cards" (see http://www.ons.org/outcomes/). 125 Enterprise Drive, RIDC Park, West Pittsburgh, PA 15275–1214 http://www.ons.org

PAIN ORGANIZATIONS FOCUSED ON CONSUMERS AND ADVOCACY

American Pain Foundation—working to improve the quality of life of people with pain by raising public awareness, providing practical information, promoting research, and advocating to remove barriers and increase access to effective pain management. Has many cutting-edge, interactive, online features (e.g., Pain-Aid, Webcasts, blogs, etc.) 201 N. Charles Street, Suite 170, Baltimore, MD 21201–4111 http://www.painfoundation.org/

American Chronic Pain Association—programs and resources to facilitate peer support, personal and family understanding, and resources to live fully despite pain. P.O. Box 850, Rocklin, CA 95677 http://www.theacpa.org

National Pain Foundation—an online educational and support community for persons in pain, their families, and physicians. Credible source for treatment options and pain information that is peer reviewed by leading pain specialists. 300 E. Hampden Avenue, Suite 100, Englewood, CO 80113 http://nationalpainfoundation.org/

National Headache Foundation—a source of reliable information and resources to help patients, families, health-care professionals, and the public. 820 N. Orleans, Suite 217, Chicago, Illinois 60610 http://www.headaches.org/

National Fibromyalgia Association—a top-quality organization with a variety of programs dedicated to improving the quality of life for people with fibromyalgia. 2121 S. Towne Centre Place, Suite 300, Anaheim, CA 92806 http://www.fmaware.org/

Cancer-Pain.org—provides accurate information and sources of support for patients with cancer pain, caregivers, and health-care professionals.

Interstitial Cystitis Association—is dedicated to helping people with interstitial cystitis, and the health-care providers and researchers to improve the lives of those with IC. 100 Park Avenue, Suite 108A, Rockville, MD 20850 http://www.ichelp.org/

The Neuropathy Association—provides support and education, advocate for patients' interests, and promotes research into the causes of and cures for neuropathy. 60 E. 42nd Street, Suite 942/New York, NY 10165 http://www.neuropathy.org/

General Sources of Information for Internet-Based Searches

SOURCE	ABOUT
National Health Information Center http://www.health.gov/NHIC	A health information referral service (for professionals and consumers) answering questions and linking to other organizations and resources.
Web MD http://www.webmd.com/	Up-to-date medical information and news. Provides a comprehensive directory of more than 4,000 diseases and conditions. Site includes message boards, newsletters, and live events.
MEDLINE http://www.ncbi.nlm.nih.gov/pubmed/	PubMed is a service of the National Library of Medicine that includes millions of citations from professional journals.
Medline Plus http://medlineplus.gov/	A searchable site with well-organized resources for the health consumer. Plain language used throughout and multilingual resources are available.

Internet-Based Pain Resources

SELECTED WEB SITES	FOCUS
Pain Management Online http://www.painmngt.com/	Commercial site for specialists in pain management. Excellent patient education resources.
Pain.Com http://www.pain.com/	An educational and informational resource on the Internet for health-care professionals and consumers who have an interest in pain and its management.
Pain Management Series www.ama-cmeonline.com	Nice current information on pain management for the professional organized in 12 modules developed and updated by the American Medical Association.
Pediatric Pain Sourcebook http://painsourcebook.ca/	Pediatric pain sourcebook provides free information, protocols, policies, and resources on pediatric pain.

Internet-Based Pain Resources—cont'd

SELECTED WEB SITES	FOCUS
Pain Treatment Topics http://pain-topics.org/	A noncommercial resource for health professionals and patients, providing open access to clinical news, information, research, and education for a better understanding of pain-management practices.
City of Hope Pain & Palliative Care Resource Center http://prc.coh.org/	An extensive clearinghouse of information and resources to improve the quality of pain management and end-of-life care. Tools facilitate pain assessment, patient education, quality assurance, and research.
Pain and Policy Study Group http://www.painpolicy.wisc.edu/	Support "balanced" laws to ensure adequate availability of pain medications for patient care while minimizing diversion and abuse. Many useful articles, tools, and state-legislation/report cards.
Mayday Pain Project http://www.painandhealth.org/	The Mayday Pain Project is an educational resource providing easily accessible, authoritative, and user-friendly information about pain care issues.
Pain Action http://www.painaction.com/	Authoritative resource that reinforces the importance of self-management for persons with chronic pain. Strategies for self-managing back pain, headache, and cancer pain are detailed.
Pain Knowledge http://www.painknowledge.org/	Authoritative, timely, comprehensive information about the assessment and management of pain for busy health-care professionals. Excellent tools, glossary, downloadable slides, and other media forms.
http://www.pain.com/	Many resources on pain for patients and professionals. Less extensive than other sites listed, but easy to navigate and reliable information.
In the Face of Pain http://www.inthefaceofpain.com/	An online kit providing tools to advocate for people in pain. Learn the basics of how to share messages about pain with community-based policy makers, media outlets, and professional organizations.
Inflexxion painACTION.com for patients PainEDU.com for professionals	Inflexxion offers a comprehensive array of opioid risk-reduction tools for professionals and helpful resources for patients with specific types of pain.

Position Papers Pertaining to Pain Management Nursing

POSITION PAPER	SPONSOR	ACCESS
Regulatory Implications of Pain Management	NCSBN	https://www.ncsbn.org/05_18_07_Pain_Statement.pdf
Management and Monitoring of Analgesia by Catheter Techniques: Position Statement	ASPMN	http://www.aspmn.org/Organization/documents/RegisteredNurseManagementandMonitoringofAnalgesiaByCatheterTechniquesPMNversion.pdf
Authorized & Unauthorized ("PCA by Proxy") Dosing: Analgesic Infusion Pumps	ASPMN	http://www.aspmn.org/Organization/documents/PMNVersionPCA.pdf
Pain Assessment in the Nonverbal Patient	ASPMN	http://www.aspmn.org/Organization/documents/NonverbalJournalFINAL.pdf
Prevention and Management of Pain in the Neonate	AAP	http://pediatrics.aappublications.org/cgi/content/full/118/5/2231 *Pediatrics, 118* (5): 2231–2241.
Assessment & Management of Acute Pain in Infants, Children, and Adolescents	AAP	http://www.cirp.org/library/pain/re9933/
Pain Management in Patients with Addictive Disease	ASPMN	http://www.aspmn.org/Organization/documents/addictions_9pt.pdf
Management of Persistent Pain in Older Persons	AGS	http://www.americangeriatrics.org/products/positionpapers/JGS5071.pdf *JAGS, 50,* S205-S224
Use of Placebos in Pain Management	ASPMN	http://www.aspmn.org/pdfs/Use%20of%20Placebos.pdf
Position Statement on Assisted Suicide	ASPMN	http://www.aspmn.org/pdfs/Assisted%20Suicide.pdf
"As-Needed" Range Orders For Opioid Analgesics to Manage Acute Pain	ASPMN	http://www.aspmn.org/pdfs/As%20Needed%20Range%20Orders.pdf
Pain Management at the End of Life	ASPMN	http://www.aspmn.org/Organization/documents/EndofLifeCare.pdf

Position Papers Pertaining to Pain Management Nursing—cont'd

POSITION PAPER	SPONSOR	ACCESS
Access To Pain Treatment (opioid medications)	United Nations	http://www.fedcp.org/news/2008082 8_statement_on_pain_treatment_and _CND_FINAL.pdf
Care Of Dying Patients	AGS	http://www.americangeriatrics.org/ products/positionpapers/careofd.shtml
Cancer Pain Management	ONS	http://www.ons.org/publications/ positions/CancerPainManagement.shtml

AAP—American Academy of Pediatrics; AGS—American Gerontological Society; NCSBN—National Council of State Boards of Nursing; ONS—Oncology Nursing Society; ASPMN—American Society for Pain Management Nursing

References
Chapter 1: The Nurse's Role in Pain Control

1. American Pain Society. (2000, January 11). *Pain assessment and treatment in the managed care environment*. Retrieved March 6, 2008 from http://www.ampainsoc.org/advocacy/assess_treat_mce.htm

2. National Institutes of Health. (1998, September 4). *NIH guide: New directions in pain research I*. Retrieved from http://grants.nih.gov/grants/guide/pa-files/PA-98-102.html

3. Martin, B. I., Deyo, R. A., Mirza, S. K., Turner, J. A., Comstock, B. A., Hollingworth, W., et al. (2008). Expenditures and health status among adults with back and neck problems. *JAMA, 299*(6), 656–664.

4. Centers for Disease Control and Prevention. (2008). *Targeting arthritis: Improving quality of life for more than 46 million Americans*. At a Glance. Retrieved March 6, 2008 from http://www.cdc.gov/nccdphp/publications/aag/arthritis.htm

5. Stewart, W. F., Ricci, J. A., Chee, E., Morganstein, D., & Lipton, R. (2003). Lost productive time and cost due to common pain conditions in the US workforce. *JAMA, 290*, 2443–2454.

6. Acute Pain Management Guideline Panel. (1992). *Acute pain management: Operative or medical procedures and trauma*. Clinical practice guideline. AHCPR Publication No. 92–0032.

7. Jacox, A., Carr, D. B., Payne, R., et al. (1994). *Management of cancer pain clinical practice guideline, No. 9*. AHCPR Publication, No. 94–0592.

8. Serlin, R. C., Mendoza, T. R., Nakamura, Y., Edwards, K. R., & Cleeland, C. S. (1995). When is cancer pain mild, moderate or severe? Grading pain severity by its interference with function. *Pain, 61*, 277–284.

9. Greipp, M. E. (1992). Undermedication for pain: An ethical model. *Advances in Nursing Science, 15*(1), 44 –53.

10. American Nurses Association. (2004). *Nursing: Scope and standards of practice.* Washington, D.C.: Nursingbooks.org

11. D'Arcy, Y., & Johann, D. (2008). Using a pain medication protocol to improve pain management. *Nursing Management, 39*(3), 35–39.

12. Mitchinson, A. R., Kim, H. M., Rosenberg, J. M., et al. (2007). Acute postoperative pain management using massage as an adjuvant_therapy: A randomized trial. *Archives of Surgery, 142*(12),1158–1167.

13. Kekkeboom, K. L., Bumpus, M., Wanta, B., & Serlin, R. C. (2008). Oncology nurses' use of nondrug pain interventions in practice. *Journal of Pain and Symptom Management, 35*(1), 83–94.

14. Bossi, L. M., Ott, M. J., & DeCristofaro, S. (2008). Reiki as a clinical intervention in oncology nursing practice. *Clinical Journal of Oncology Nursing, 12*(3), 489–494.

15. Loeser, J. D., Seres, J. L., & Newman, R. I. (1990). Interdisciplinary, multimodal management of chronic pain. In J.J. Bonica, *The management of pain* (2nd ed.,Vol. I). Philadelphia: Lea and Febiger.

16. Salerno, E., & Willens, J. S. (1996). *Pain management handbook: An interdisciplinary approach.* St. Louis: Mosby Year Book.

17. Burckhardt, M. A., & Nathaniel, A. K. (2008). *Ethics and issues in contemporary nursing* (3rd ed.). Thomson Delmar Learning.

18. Kirk, T. (2002). Managing pain, managing ethics. *Pain Management Nursing, 8*(1), 25–34.

19. Vaglienti, C.S., & Grinberg, M. (2004). Emerging liability for the undertreatment of pain. *Journal of Nursing Law, 9,* 7–18.

20. Shapiro, R. S. (1996). Health care providers' liability exposure for inappropriate pain management. *Journal of Law and Medical Ethics, 24*(4), 360–364.

21. Rich, B. A. (2003). A placebo for the pain: A medico-legal case analysis. *Pain Medicine, 4*(4), 366–372.

22. American Society for Pain Management Nursing and American Nurses Association. (2005). *Pain management nursing: Scope and standards of practice.* Silver Spring, MD: Nursingbooks.org

23. Paice, J. A., Barnard, C., Creamer, J., & Omerod, K. (2006). Creating organizational change through the pain resource nurse program. *Joint Commission Journal on Quality and Patient Safety, 32*(1), 24–31.

24. Berry, P. H., & Dahl, J. L. (2007). Advanced practice nurse controlled substances prescriptive authority: A review of the regulations and implications for effective pain management at end-of-life. *Journal of Hospice and Palliative Care Nursing, 9*(5), 238–245.

Chapter 2: The Nature of Pain

1. National Center for Health Statistics Health, United States. (2006). *Chartbook on trends in the health of Americans.* Retrieved April 24, 2008 from http://www.cdc.gov/nchs/data/hus/hus06.pdf

2. Stewart, W. F., Ricci, J. A., Chee, E., et al. (2003). Lost productive time and cost due to common pain conditions in the U.S. workforce. *JAMA, 290,* 2443–2454.

3. Rivara, F. P., Mackenzie, E.J., Jurkovich, G.J., et al. (2008). Prevalence of pain in patients 1 year after major trauma. *Archives of Surgery, 143*(3),282–287.

4. Gerstle, D. S., All, A. C., & Wallace, D. C. (2001). Quality of life and chronic nonmalignant pain. *Pain Management Nursing, 2*(3), 98–109.

5. Mersky, H., Loesser, J. D., & Dubner, R. (2005). *The paths of pain*. Seattle: IASP Press.

6. Melzack, R., & Wall, P. D. (1983). *The Challenge of Pain*. New York: Basic Books.

7. Arnstein, P. M. (2002). Theories of pain. In B. St. Marie (Ed.), *Core curriculum for pain management nurses* (pp. 107–119). Philadelphia: W.B. Saunders Co.

8. Cairns, D. M., Adkins, R. H., & Scott, M. D. (1996). Pain and depression in acute traumatic spinal cord injury: Origins of chronic problematic pain? *Archives of Physical Medicine and Rehabilitation, 77*, 329–335.

9. Magni, G., Moreschi, C., Rigatti-Luchini, S., & Merskey, H. (1994). Prospective study on the relationship between depressive symptoms and chronic musculoskeletal pain. *Pain, 56*, 289–297.

10. Melzack, R., & Wall, P. D. (1965). Pain mechanisms: A new theory. *Science, 150*, 971–979.

11. Merskey, H., & Bogduk, N. (Eds). (1994). Pain terms: A current list with definitions and notes on usage. In *Classification of chronic pain* (2nd ed., pp. 209–214). IASP Task Force on Taxonomy. Seattle: IASP Press.

12. International Headache Society. (2004). *The international headache classification (ICHD-2)*. Retrieved May 7, 2008 from http://ihs-classification.org/en/

13. Serlin, R. C., Mendoza, T. R., Nakamura, et al. (1995). When is cancer pain mild, moderate or severe? Grading pain severity by its interference with function. *Pain, 61*(2), 277–284.

14. North American Nursing Diagnosis Association. (2007). NANDA *nursing diagnosis: Definitions and classifications* (7th ed.). Philadelphia: NANDA International.

15. Kehlet, H., Jensen, T. S., & Woolf, C. J. (2007). Persistent postsurgical pain: Risk factors and prevention. *Lancet, 13*,367(9522), 1618–1625.

16. Perkins, F. M., & Kehlet, H. (2000). Chronic pain as an outcome of surgery: A review of predictive factors. *Anesthesiology, 93*, 1123–1133.

17. Reuben, S. S., & Buvanendran, A. (2007). Preventing the development of chronic pain after orthopedic surgery with preventive multimodal analgesia techniques. *The Journal of Bone and Joint Surgery, 89*, 1343–1358.

18. Macrae, W. A. (2001). Chronic pain after surgery. *British Journal of Anaesthesia, 87*(1), 88–98.

19. Bernabei, R., Gambassi, G., Lapane, K., et al. (1998). Management of pain in elderly patients with cancer. SAGE study group. Systematic: Systematic assessment of geriatric drug use via epidemiology. *JAMA, 279*, 1877–1882.

20. McMahon, S. B., & Koltzenberg, M. (Eds.). (2006). Neurobiology of pain. In Wall and Melzack's Textbook of pain (pp. 3–218). London: Elsevier Churchill Livingstone.

21. Melzack, R. (2001). Pain and the neuromatrix in the brain. *Journal of Dental Education, 65*(12), 1378–1382.

22. Wall, P. (1999). *Pain: The science of suffering*. London: Weidenfeld & Nicolson (Orion) Publishing.

23. Edwards, R. R., Almieda, D. M., Klick, B., et al. (2008). Duration of sleep contributes to next-day pain report in the general population. *Pain,* (Epub ahead of print).

24. American Academy of Pediatrics and American Pain Society. (2001). The assessment and management of acute pain in infants, children and adolescents. *Pediatrics, 108* (3), 793.

25. Kabat-Zinn, J. (1994). *Wherever you go, there you are: Mindfulness meditation in everyday life.* New York: Hyperion.

26. Arnstein, P., Caudill, M., Mandle, C. L., et al. (1999). Self-efficacy as a mediator of the relationship between pain intensity, disability and depression in chronic pain patients. *Pain, 80*(3), 483–491.

27. McCracken, L. M. (2005). Social context and acceptance of chronic pain: The role of solicitous and punishing responses. *Pain, 113*(1–2),155–159.

28. Flor, H., Breitenstein, C., Birbaumer, N., et al. (2000). A psychophysiological analysis of spouse solicitousness towards pain behaviors, spouse interaction, and pain perception. *Behavioral Therapy, 26*(2), 255–272.

29. De Good, D. E., & Kiernan, B. D. (1997). Pain related cognitions as predictors of pain treatment outcomes. *Advances in Medical Psychotherapy, 9,* 73–90.

30. Arnstein, P. M., Wells-Federman, C., & Caudill-Slosberg, M. A. (2002, August). Change in self-efficacy as a predictor of clinical outcomes and coping skill use at one year following participation in a cognitive behavioral pain treatment program (Poster presentation, 10th World Congress on Pain in San Diego CA). Seattle, WA: International Association for the Study of Pain (IASP).

31. McCracken, L. M. (1998). Learning to live with the pain: Acceptance of pain predicts adjustment in persons with chronic pain. *Pain, 74,* 21–27.

32. Atkin, K. (2000). Adults with disabilities who report excellent or good quality of life had established a balance of body, mind, and spirit. *Evidence Based Nursing, 3*(1), 31.

33. Jacob, M. C., & Kerns, R. D. (2001). Assessment of the psychosocial context of the experience of chronic pain. In D. C. Turk, R. Melzack (Eds.), *Handbook of pain assessment* (2nd ed., pp. 362–384). New York: The Guilford Press.

34. Ang, D. C., Peloso, P. M., Woolson, R. F., et al. (2006). Predictors of incident chronic widespread pain among veterans following the first Gulf War. *Clinical Journal of Pain, 22*(6), 554–563.

35. Laurell, K., Larsson, B., & Eeg-Olofsson, O. (2005). Headache in schoolchildren: Association with other pain, family history and psychosocial factors. *Pain, 119*(1–3), 150–158.

36. Bergman, S. (2005). Psychosocial aspects of chronic widespread pain and fibromyalgia. *Disability & Rehabilitation, 27*(12), 675–683.

37. Fillingim, R. B., Edwards, R. R., & Powell, T. (2000). Sex-dependent effects of reported familial pain history on recent pain complaints and experimental pain responses. *Pain, 86*(1–2), 87–94.

38. Walsh, C. A., Jamieson, E., Macmillan, H., & Boyle, M. (2007). Child abuse and chronic pain in a community survey of women. *Journal of Interpersonal Violence, 22*(12), 1536–1554.

39. Sachs-Ericsson, N., Kendall-Tackett, K., & Hernandez, A. (2007). Childhood abuse, chronic pain, and depression in the national comorbidity survey. *Child Abuse & Neglect, 31*(5), 531–547.

40. Wells-Federman, C. L. (2000). Care of the patient with chronic pain: Part II. *Clinical Excellence for Nurse Practitioners, 4*(1), 4–12.

41. Arnstein, P. M., Vidal, M., Wells-Federman, C., et al. (2002). From chronic pain patient to peer: Benefits and risks of volunteering. *Pain Management Nursing, 3*(3), 94–103.

42. Sherman, R., & Hickner, J. (2008). Academic physicians use placebos in clinical practice and believe in the mind-body connection. *Journal of General and Internal Medicine, 23*(1), 7–10.

43. Greipp, M. E. (1992). Undermedication for pain: An ethical model. *Advances in Nursing Science, 15*(1), 44–53.

44. Kolcaba, K., Tilton, C., & Drouin, C. (2006). Comfort theory: A unifying framework to enhance the practice environment. *Journal of Nursing Administration, 36* (11), 538–544.

45. Dodd, M. J., Janson, S., Facione, N., et al. (2001). Advancing the science of symptom management. *Journal of Advanced Nursing, 33* (5), 668–676.

46. Good, M. (1998). A middle-range theory of acute pain management: Use in research. *Nursing Outlook, 46*(3), 120–124.

Chapter 3: Physiology of Pain

1. Arnstein, P. M. (2003). Understanding pain. In J. Munden (Ed.), *Pain management made incredibly easy* (pp. 1–28). Philadelphia: Lippincott Williams & Wilkins.

2. Yaksh, T. L. (2008). A review of pain processing pharmacology. In H. T. Benzon, J. P. Rathmell, C. L., Wu, D. C., Turk, C. E., & Argoff (Eds.), *Raj's practical management of pain* (4th ed., pp. 135–149). St. Louis, Mosby.

3. Yaksh, T. L. (2007). Dynamics of the pain processing system. In S. D. Waldman (Ed.), *Pain management* (pp. 21–31). Philadelphia: Saunders Elsevier Publishers.

4. Edwards, A. D. (2002). Physiology of pain. In B. St. Marie (Ed.), *Core curriculum for pain management nurses* (pp. 121–145). Philadelphia: W.B. Saunders Co.

5. Apkarian, A. V. (2008). Pain and brain changes. In H. T. Benzon, J. P. Rathmell, C. L. Wu, D. C. Turk & C. E. Argoff (Eds.), *Raj's practical management of pain* (4th ed., pp. 151–169). St. Louis: Mosby.

6. Melzack, R., & Wall, P. D. (1982). *The challenge of pain.* New York: Basic Books.

7. Liu, L. M., Hu, D. Y., Pan, X. K., et al. (2005). Subclass opioid receptors associated with the cardiovascular depression after traumatic shock and the antishock effects of its specific receptor antagonists. *Shock, 24*(5), 470–475.

8. Ballantyne, J. C., Carr, D. B., deFerranti, S., et al. (1998). The comparative effects of postoperative analgesic therapies on pulmonary outcomes: cumulative meta-analyses of randomized controlled trials. *Anesthesia and Analgesia, 86,* 598–612.

9. Acute Pain Management Guideline Panel. (1992). *Acute pain management: Operative or medical procedures and trauma.* Clinical Practice Guideline. AHCPR Publication No. 92–0032.

10. Pavlin, D. J., Cen, C., Penaloza, D. A., et al. (2002). Pain as a factor complicating recovery and discharge alter ambulatory surgery. *Anesthesia and Analgesia, 95,* 627–634.

11. Elsenbruch, S., Haag, S., Lucas, A., et al. (2007). Neuroendocrine and blood pressure responses to rectal distensions in individuals with high and low visceral pain sensitivity. *Psychoneuroendocrinology, 32*(5), 580–585.

12. Greisen, J., Juhl, C. B., Grofte, T., et al. (2001). Acute pain induces insulin resistance in humans. *Anesthesiology, 95,* 578–584.

13. Lvungqvist, O., Nygren, J., Soop, M., et al. (2006). Metabolic postoperative management: novel concepts. *Current Opinion in Critical Care, 11,* 295–299.

14. Page, G. G., Ben-Eliyahu, S., Yirmiya, R., & Liebeskind, J. C. (1993). Morphine attenuates surgery-induced enhancement of metastatic colonization in rats. *Pain, 54*(1), 21–28.

15. Rittner, H. L., Brack, A., & Stein, C. (2008). Pain and the immune system. *British Journal of Anesthesia, 101*(1), 40–44.

16. Desai, P. M. (1999). Pain management and pulmonary dysfunction. *Critical Care Clinics, 15* (1), 151–166.

17. Perkins, F. M., & Kehlet, H. (2000). Chronic pain as an outcome of surgery. *Anesthesiology, 93,* 1123–1133.

18. Macrae, W. A. (2001). Chronic pain after surgery. *British Journal of Anesthesia, 87,* 88–93.

19. Macrae, W. A. (2008). Chronic post-surgical pain: 10 years on. *British Journal of Anesthesia, 101*(1), 77–86.

20. Grass, P. (2000). The role of epidural anesthesia and analgesia in postoperative outcomes. *Regional Anesthesia, 18,* 407–428.

21. Arnstein, P. M. (1997). The neuroplastic phenomenon: A physiologic link between chronic pain and learning. *Journal of Neuroscience Nursing, 29*(3), 179–186.

22. Mitchell, A., & Boss, B. J. (2002). Adverse effects of pain on the nervous system of newborns and young children: A review of the literature. *Journal of Neuroscience Nursing, 34*(5), 228–236.

23. Woolf, C. J., & Salter, M. W. (2000) Neuronal plasticity: Increasing the gain in pain. *Science, 288,* 1765–1768.

24. Cohen, S. A. (2004). Pathophysiology of pain. In C. A. Warfield & Z. H. Bajwa (Eds.), *Principles and practice of pain medicine* (2nd ed., pp. 35–43). New York: McGraw Hill.

25. Mao, J., & Mayer, D. J. (2001). Spinal cord neuroplasticity following repeated exposure and its relation to pathological pain. *Annals of New York Academy of Science, 933,* 175–184.

26. DuPen, A., Shen, D., & Ersek, M. (2007). Mechanisms of opioid-induced tolerance and hyperalgesia. *Pain Management Nursing, 8*(3), 113–121.

27. Polgar, E., Hughes, D. I., Riddel, J. S., et al. (2003). Selective loss of spinal GABAergic or glycinergic neurons is not necessary for development of thermal hyperalgesia in the chronic constriction injury model of neuropathic pain. *Pain,* 104, 229–291.

28. Woolf, C. J., Shortland, P., & Coggeshall, R. E. (1992). Peripheral nerve injury triggers central sprouting of myelinated afferents. *Nature, 355,* 75–78.

29. Maciver, K., Lloyd, D. M., Kelly, S., et al. (2008). Phantom limb pain, cortical reorganization and the therapeutic effects of mental imagery. *Brain, 131*(8), 2181–2191.

29a. McLachlap, et al. (1993). Peripheral nerve injury triggers noradrenergic sprouting within dorsal root ganglia. *Nature, 363,* 543–546.

30. Kramer, H. H., Stenner, C., Seddigh, S., Bauermann, T., Birklein, F., Maihofer, C. (2008). Illusion of Pain: Pre-existing knowledge determines brain activation of imagined allodynia. *Journal of Pain, 9*(6), 543–551.

31. Mao, J. (2008). Opioid-induced hyperalgesia. *Pain Clinical Updates,16*(2), 1–4.

Chapter 4: Pain Assessment

1. Arnstein, P. M. (2003). Comprehensive analysis and management of chronic pain. *Nursing Clinics of North America, 38,* 403–417.

2. Carr, D. B., Reines, H. D., Schaffer, J., Polomano, R. C., & Lande, S. (2005). The impact of technology on the analgesic gap and quality of acute pain management. *Regional Anesthesia & Pain Medicine, 30*(3), 286–291.

3. Payne, R. (2000). Chronic pain: Challenges in the assessment and management of cancer pain. *Journal of Pain and Symptom Management, 19*(1 Suppl.), S12–S15.

4. The Joint Commission. (2009). *Comprehensive accreditation manual: The e-edition.* Oakbrook Terrace, IL. Retrieved January 22, 2009 from http://e-edition.jcrinc.com

5. McCaffery, M., & Pasero, C. (1999). *Pain: Clinical manual* (2nd ed.). St. Louis, Mosby.

6. Jensen, M. T., & Petersen, K. L. (2006). Gender differences in pain and secondary hyperalgesia after heat/capsaicin sensitization in healthy volunteers. *Journal of Pain*, 7(3), 211–217.

7. Edwards, C. L., Fillingim, R. B., & Keefe, F. (2001). Race, ethnicity and pain. *Pain.* 94(2), 133–7

8. American Nurses Association (ANA) and American Society for Pain Management Nursing (ASPMN). (2005) *Pain management nursing: Scope and standards of practice* (p. 11). Silver Spring, MD: ANA.

9. Fink, R. (2000). Pain assessment: The cornerstone to optimal pain management. *Baylor University Medical Center Proceedings, 13*(3), 236–239.

10. Gordon, D. B., Dahl, J. L., Miaskowski, C., McCarberg, B., Todd, K. H., Paice, J. A., et al. (2005). American Pain Society recommendations for improving the quality of acute and cancer pain management. *Archives of Internal Medicine, 165*, 1574–1580.

11. Gloth, F. M. III, Scheve, A. A., Stober, C. V., Chow, S., & Prosser, J. (2001). The functional pain scale: Reliability, validity and responsiveness in an elderly population. *Journal of the American Medical Directors Association, 2*(3), 110–114.

12. DeGowin, R. L., & Brown, D. D. (2000). *DeGowin's diagnostic examination* (7th ed.). New York: McGraw-Hill.

13. McMahon, S. B., & Kolzenberg, M. (Eds.). (2006). *Wall and Melzack's textbook of pain* (5th ed., pp. 291–317). Philadelphia: Elsevier Churchill Livingstone.

14. Institute for Safe Medication Practices. (2002). Pain scales don't weigh every risk. *ISMP Medication Safety Alert! Acute Care, 7*(15), 1–2.

15. American Academy of Pediatrics and Canadian Paediatric Society. (2006). Policy statement: Prevention and management of pain in the neonate: An update. *Pediatrics, 118* (5), 2231–2241.

16. Breau, L. M., McGrath, P. J., Craig, K. D., Santor, D., Cassidy, K. L., & Reid, G. J. (2001). Facial expression of children receiving immunizations: A principal components analysis of the child facial coding system. *Clinical Journal of Pain, 17*(2), 178–186.

17. Grunnau, R. V. E., & Craig, K. D. (1987). Pain expression in neonates: Facial action and cry. *Pain, 28*, 395–410.

18. Anand, K. J. S., Aranda, J. V., Berde, C. B., Buckman, S., Capparelli, E. V., Carlo, W., et al. (2006). Summary proceedings from the neonatal pain-control group. *Pediatrics, 117*(3), S9–S22.

19. Malviya, S., Voepel-Lewis, T., Burke, C., Merkel, S. I., & Tait, A. R. (2006). The revised FLACC observational pain tool: improved reliability and validity for pain assessment in children with cognitive impairment. *Pediatric Anesthesia, 16*, 258–265.

20. Manworren, R. C. B., & Hynan, L. S. (2003). Practice applications of research. Clinical validation of FLACC: Preverbal patient pain scale. *Pediatric Nursing, 29*(2), 140–146.

21. Finley, G. A., & McGrath, P. J. (1998). Measurement of pain in infants and children. *Progress in pain research and management* (Vol. 10). Seattle: IASP Press.

22. CDC Reports Center for Disease Control. (2006). *Health, United States, 2006 with chartbook on trends in the health of Americans.* Hyattsville, MD: U.S. Government Printing Office #76-641496. Retrieved September 21, 2007 from http://www.cdc.gov/nchs/data/hus/hus06.pdf

23. American Geriatrics Society. (2002). AGS panel on persistent pain in older persons. Clinical practice guidelines: The management of persistent pain in older persons. *Journal of the American Geriatrics Society, 50*, S205–S224.

24. Herr, K., Bjoro, K., & Decker, S. (2006). Tools for assessment of pain in non-verbal older adults with dementia: A state-of-the-science review. *Journal of Pain and Symptom Management, 31*(2), 170–192.

25. Warden, V., Hurley, A. C., & Volicer, L. (2003). Development and psychometric evaluation of the pain assessment in advanced dementia (PAINAD) scale. *Journal of the American Medical Directors Association, 4*(1), 9–15.

26. Herr, K., Coyne, P. J., Key, T., Manworren, R., McCaffery, M., Merkel, S., et al. (2006). Pain assessment in the nonverbal patient: position statement with clinical practice recommendations. *Pain Management Nursing, 7*(2), 44–52.

27. Payen, J. F., Bru, O., Bosson, J. L., Lagrasta, A., Novel, E., Deschaux, I., et al. (2001). Assessing pain in critically ill sedated patients using a behavioral pain scale. *Critical Care Medicine, 29*(12), 2258–2263.

28. Gelinas, C., Fillion, L., Puntillo, K., Viens, C., & Fortier, M. (2006). Validation of the critical-care pain observation tool in adult patients. *American Journal of Critical Care, 15* (24), 420–427.

29. Von Korff, M., Ormel, J., Keefe, F. J., & Dworkin, S. F. (1992). Grading the severity of chronic pain. *Pain, 50*, 133–149.

30. McCaffery, M., Grimm, M. A., Pasero, C., Ferrell, B., & Uman, G. C. (2005). On the meaning of "drug seeking." *Pain Management Nursing, 6*(4), 122–136.

31. Weissman, D. E., & Haddox, J. D. (1989). Opioid pseudoaddiction: An iatrogenic syndrome. *Pain, 36*, 363–366.

32. Jamison, R. N., Kauffman, J., & Katz, N. P. (2000). Characteristics of methadone maintenance patients with chronic pain. *Journal of Pain and Symptom Management, 19*(1), 53–62.

33. Morgan, B. (2006). Knowing how to play the game: Hospitalized substance abusers' strategies for obtaining pain relief. *Pain Management Nursing, 7*(1), 31–41.

33a. American Academy of Pain Medicine, American Pain Society, and American Society of Addiction Medicine. Definitions Related to the Use of Opioids for the Treatment of Pain. Glenview, IL, American Academy of Pain Medicine, 2001.

34. Brown, R.L., & Rounds, L.A. (1995). Conjoint screening questionnaires for alcohol and drug abuse. *Wisconsin Medical Journal, 94*, 135–140.

35. Akbik, H., Butler, S. F., Budman, S. H., Fernandez, K., Katz, N. P., & Jamison, R. N. (2006). Validation and clinical application of the screener and opioids assessment for patients with pain (SOAPP). *Journal of Pain and Symptom Management, 32*, 287–293.

36. Butler, S. F., Budman, S. H., Fernandez, K. C., Houle, B., Benoit, C., Katz, N. P., et al. (2007). Development and validation of the current opioid misuse measure. *Pain 130*, 144–156.

37. Narcessian, E. J., & Yoon, H. J. (1997). False-positive urine drug screen: Beware the poppy seed bagel. *Journal of Pain and Symptom Management, 14*(5), 261–263.

38. American Society for Pain Management Nursing. (2005). *Position statement: Pain management in patients with addictive disease.* Retrieved September 24, 2007 from http://www.aspmn.org/pdfs/Addictive%20Disease.pdf

39. American Nurses Association. (2003). *Nursing's social policy statement* (2nd ed.). Washington, DC: American Nurses Association.

Chapter 5: Diagnoses, Treatment Planning, and Refinement

1. Gordon, M. (2007). *Manual of Nursing Diagnosis* (11th ed., pp. 229–227). Sudbury, MA: Jones & Bartlett Publishers.

2. Moorhead, S., Johnson, M., Maas, M., & Swanson E. (2008). *Nursing Outcomes Classification* (4th ed.). St. Louis, MO: Mosby Elsevier.

3. Martin, P. R. (2001). How do trigger factors acquire the capacity to precipitate headaches? *Behaviour Research and Therapy, 39* (65), 545–554.

4. Martin, P. R., Reece, J., & Forsyth, M. (2006). Noise as a trigger for headaches: Relationship between exposure and sensitivity. *Headache, 46* (6), 962–972.

5. Breau, L. M., Finley, G. A., McGrath, P. J., et al. (2002). Validation of the non-communicating children's pain checklist post-operative version. *Anesthesiology, 96* (3), 528–535.

6. Paice, J. A., Noskin, G. A., Vanagunas, A., & Shott S. (2005). Efficacy and safety of scheduled dosing of opioid analgesics: A quality improvement study. *Journal of Pain, 6* (10), 639–643.

7. American Society for Pain Management Nursing and American Nurses Association. (2005). *Pain management nursing: Scope and standards of practice.* Silver Spring, MD: Nursingbooks.org

8. Caudill, M. A. (2002). *Managing pain before it manages you* (Rev. ed.). New York: Guilford Press.

9. ReliefInsite. (2008). *Keeping a diary provides control and aids in treatment.* Retrieved September 1, 2008 from http://www.reliefinsite.com/users

10. Gaertner, J., Elsner, F., Pollmann-Dahmen, K., et al. (2004). Electronic pain diary: A randomized crossover study. *Journal of Pain and Symptom Management, 28*, 259–267.

11. American Academy of Pediatrics and Canadian Paediatric Society. (2006). Policy statement: Prevention and management of pain in the neonate: An Update. *Pediatrics, 118* (5), 2231–2241.

12. MacLean, S., Obispo, J., & Young, K. D. (2007). The gap between pediatric emergency department procedural pain management treatments available and actual practice. *Pediatric Emergency Care, 23*(2), 87–93.

13. Looi, Y., & Audisio, R. (2007). A review of the literature on post-operative pain in older cancer patients. *European Journal of Cancer, 43*(15), 2222–2230.

14. Liem, E. B., Lin, C. M., Suleman, M. I., et al. (2004). Anesthetic requirement is increased in redheads. *Anesthesiology, 101*(2), 279–283.

15. Mogil, J. S., Ritchie, J., & Smith, S. B. (2005). Melanocortin-1 receptor gene variants affect pain and μ-opioid analgesia in mice and humans. *Journal of Medical Genetics, 42*, 583–587.

16. Cepeda, M. S., & Carr, D. B. (2003). Women experience more pain and require more morphine than men to achieve a similar degree of analgesia. *Anesthesia & Analgesia, 97*, 1464–1468.

17. Greenspan, J. D., Craft, R. M., LeResche, L., et al. (2007). Studying sex and gender differences in pain and analgesia: A consensus report. *Pain, 132*(Suppl. 1), S26–S45.

18. Miners, J. O., Grgurinovich, N., Whitehead, A. G., et al. (1986). Influence of gender and oral contraceptive steroids on the metabolism of salicylic acid and acetylsalicylic acid. *British Journal of Clinical Pharmacology, 22*, 135–142.

19. Bijur, P. E., Esses, D., Birnbaum, A., et al. (2008). Responses to morphine in male and female patients: Analgesia and adverse events. *Clinical Journal of Pain, 24*, 192–198.

20. Cotreau, M. M., von Moltke, L. L., & Breenblatt, D. L. (2005). The influence of age and sex on clearance of cytochrome P450 3A substrates. *Clinical Pharmacokinetics, 44*, 33–60.

21. Zacny, J. P., & Beckman, N. J. (2004). The effects of cold water stimulus on butorphanol effects in males and females. *Pharmacology Biochemistry and Behavior, 78*, 653–659.

22. Walker, J. S., & Carmody, J. J. (1998). Experimental pain in healthy human subjects: Gender differences in nociception and in response to ibuprofen. *Anesthesia & Analgesia, 86*, 1257–1262.

23. Strickland, J. W. (1998). Considerations for the treatment of the injured athlete. *Clinics in Sports Medicine, 17*(3), 397–400.

24. Light, D. Transcultural nursing care: Middle eastern community. *Transcultural Nursing* Web site. Retrieved January 27, 2009 from http://www.culturediversity.org/mide.htm

25. Bandura, A. (1997). *Self-efficacy: The exercise of control.* NY: W. H. Freeman and Company.

26. Arnstein, P. M., Caudill, M. A., Wells-Federman, C. (2000). Self-efficacy as a mediator of depression and pain-related disability in chronic pain. In M. Devor, M. Rowbotham & Z. Wiesenfeld-Hallin (Eds.), *Progress in pain research and management* (Vol. 16, pp.1105–1111). Seattle: IASP Press.

27. Shelby, R. A., Somers, T. J., Keefe, F. J., et al. (2008). Domain specific self-efficacy mediates the impact of pain catastrophizing on pain and disability in overweight and obese osteoarthritis patients. *Journal of Pain, 9*(10), 912–919.

28. Resnick, B., Luisi, D., & Vogel, A. (2008). Testing the senior exercise self-efficacy project (SESEP) for use with urban dwelling minority older adults. *Public Health Nursing, 25*(3), 221–234.

1. Food and Drug Administration (FDA). (2007, May 5). *FDA announces important changes and additional warnings for COX-2 selective and non-selective non-steroidal anti-inflammatory drugs (NSAIDs)*. Retrieved March 28, 2008 from http://www.fda.gov/cder/drug/advisory/COX2.htm

2. Institute for Safe Medication Practices (ISMP). (2008). *ISMP's list of high-alert medications*. Retrieved March 28, 2008 from http://www.ismp.org/tools/highalertmedications.pdf

3. WHO. (1996). *Cancer pain relief with a guide to opioid availability*. Geneva WHO Press. Retrieved from http://whqlibdoc.who.int/publications/9241544821.pdf

4. American Pain Society (APS). (2008). *Principles of analgesic use in the treatment of acute pain and cancer pain* (6th ed.). Glenview, IL: APS Press.

5. Foley, K. M. (2006). *Appraising the WHO analgesic ladder on its 20th anniversary*. Retrieved March 25, 2008 from http://www.whocancerpain.wisc.edu/old_site/eng/19_1/Interview.html

6. Paice, J. A., Noskin, G. A., Vanagunas, A., & Shott, S. (2005). Efficacy and safety of scheduled dosing of opioid analgesics: A quality improvement study. *Journal of Pain, 6* (10), 639–643.

7. Green, R., Bulloch, B., Kabani, A., Hancock, B. J., & Tenenbein, M. (2005). Early analgesia for children with acute abdominal pain. *Pediatrics, 116*(4), 978–983.

8. Attard, A. R., Corlett, M. J., Kidner, N. J., Leslie, A. P., & Fraser, I. A. (1992). Safety of early pain relief for acute abdominal pain. *British Medical Journal, 305*, 554–556.

9. Pace, S., & Burke, T. F. (1996). Intravenous morphine for early pain relief in patients with acute abdominal pain. *Academy of Emergency Medicine, 3*, 1086–1092.

10. LoVecchio, F., Oster, N., Sturmann, K., Nelso, L. S., Flashner, S., & Finger, R. (1997). The use of analgesics in patients with acute abdominal pain. *Journal of Emergency Medicine, 15*, 775–779.

11. Wolfe, J. M., Lein, D. Y., Lenkoski, K., Smithline, H. A. (2000). Analgesic administration to patients with an acute abdomen: A survey of emergency medicine physicians. *American Journal of Emergency Medicine, 18*, 250–253.

12. Vermeulen, B., Morabia, A., Unger, P. F., Goehring, C., Skljarov, I., & Terrier, F. (1999). Acute appendicitis: Influence of early pain relief on the accuracy of clinical and US findings in the decision to operate—a randomized trial. *Radiology, 210*, 639–643.

13. Frei, S. P., Bond, W. F., Bazuro, R. K., et al. (2008). Is early analgesia associated with delayed treatment of appendicitis? *American Journal of Emergency Medicine, 26*, 176–180.

14. Dionne, R. (2000). Preemptive vs. preventive analgesia: Which approach improves clinical outcomes? *Compendium of Continuing Education in Dentistry, 21*(1), 48, 51–54, 56.

15. Sun, T., Sacan, O., White, P. F., et al. (2008). Perioperative versus postoperative celecoxib on patient outcomes after major plastic surgery procedures. *Anesthesia & Analgesia, 106*, 950–958.

16. Truini, A., & Cruccu, G. (2006). Pathophysiological mechanisms of neuropathic pain. *Journal of the Neurological Sciences, 27(Suppl.)*2, S179–S182.

17. Dworkin, R. H., Connor, A. B., Backonja, M., Farrar, J. T., Finnerup, N. B., Jensen, T. S., et al. (2007). Pharmacologic management of neuropathic pain: Evidence-based recommendations. *Pain, 132*, 237–251.

18. Wunsch, M. J., Stanard, V., & Schnoll, S. H. (2003). Treatment of pain in pregnancy. *Clinical Journal of Pain, 19*(3), 148–155.

19. Griffin, M. R. (1998). Epidemiology of nonsteroidal anti-inflammatory drug-associated gastrointestinal injury. *American Journal of Medicine, 104*(3A), 23S–29S.

20. Ong, C. K. S., Lirk, P., Tan, C.H., & Seymour, R. A. (2007). An evidence-based update on nonsteroidal anti-inflammatory drugs. *Clinical Medicine and Research, 5*(1), 19–34.

21. Anaokar, S. M., Parulekar, S. V., Thatte, U. M., & Dahanukar, S. A. (1993). A multiple dose comparison of ketorolac tromethamine with ibuprofen for analgesic activity. *Journal of Postgraduate Medicine, 39*:74.

22. Novak D., Lewis, J. (2003). Drug-induced liver disease. *Current Opinion in Gastroenterology, 19*(3), 203–215.

23. Miaskowski, C., Cleary, J., Burney, R., Coyne, P., Finley, R., Foster, R., et al. (2005). *Guideline for the management of cancer pain in adults and children.* APS Clinical Practice Guideline Series, No. 3. Glenview, IL: American Pain Society.

24. Moryl, N., Coyle, N., Foley, K. M. (2008). Managing an acute pain crisis in a patient with advanced cancer. *JAMA, 299*(12), 1457–1467.

Chapter 7: Nondrug, Complementary, and Alternative Medicine Approaches to Pain Relief

1. American Medical Association. (2007). *Module 2 pain management: Overview of management options* (pp. 1–19). Chicago, IL: American Medical Association.

2. Barnes, P. M., Powell-Griner E., McFann, K., et al. (2004). Complementary and alternative medicine use among adults: United States, 2002. *Advance Data, 343*, 1–19.

3. Eisenberg, D. M., Davis, R. B., Ettner, S. L. (1998). Trends in alternative medicine use in the United States, 1990–1997: Results of a follow-up national survey. *JAMA, 280*(18), 1569–1575.

4. Panel on Definition and Description. (1997). CAM research methodology conference. Defining and describing complementary and alternative medicine. *Alternative Therapies in Health & Medicine, 3*(2), 49–57.

5. National Center for Complementary and Alternative Medicine. (2007). Use of CAM in the United States. Retrieved October 13, 2008 from http://nccam.nih.gov/news/camuse.pdf

6. Saper, R. B., Phillips, R. S., Sehgal, A., Khouri, N., et al. (2008). Lead, mercury, and arsenic in U.S.- and Indian-manufactured Ayurvedic medicines sold via the internet. *JAMA, 300*(8), 915–923.

7. Koh, H. L., & Woo, S. O. (2000). Chinese proprietary medicine in Singapore: Regulatory control of toxic heavy metals and undeclared drugs. *Drug Safety, 23*(5), 351–362.

8. Shang, A., Huwiler-Müntener, K., Nartey, L., et al. (2005). "Are the clinical effects of homoeopathy placebo effects? Comparative study of placebo-controlled trials of homoeopathy and allopathy." *Lancet, 366*(9487), 726–732.

9. Pittler, M. H., & Ernst, E. (2008). Complementary therapies for neuropathic and neuralgic pain: A systematic review. *Clinical Journal of Pain, 24*(8), 731–733.

10. Arnstein, P. M., Wells-Federman, C., & Caudill-Slosberg, M. A. (2002). *Change in self-efficacy as a predictor of clinical outcomes and coping skill use at one year following participation in a cognitive behavioral pain treatment program.* Poster presentation, 10th World Congress on Pain in San Diego, CA. Seattle, WA: International Association for the Study of Pain (IASP).

11. Caudill, M. A., Schnable, R., Zuttermeister, P., et al. (1991). Decreased clinic use by chronic pain patients: Response to behavioral medicine intervention. *Clinical Journal of Pain, 7*, 305–310.

12. Moore, J. E., Von Korff, M., Cherkin, D., et al. (2000). A randomized trial of a cognitive-behavioral program for enhancing back pain self care in a primary care setting. *Pain, 88*, 145–153.

13. Wells-Federman, C., Arnstein, P. M., & Caudill-Slosberg, M. A. (2002). Nurse-led pain-management program: Effect on self-efficacy, pain intensity, pain-related disability and depressive symptoms in chronic pain patients. *Pain Management Nursing, 3*(5), 141–153.

14. Towheed, T. E., Maxwell, L., Anastassiades, T.P., et al. (2005). Glucosamine therapy for treating osteoarthritis. *Cochrane Database of Systematic Reviews* 2005, Issue 2, Art. No. CD002946.

15. Cherkin, D. C., Sherman, K. J., Deyo, R. A., et al. (2003). A review of the evidence for the effectiveness, safety, and cost of acupuncture, massage therapy, and spinal manipulation for back pain. *Annals of Internal Medicine, 138*(11), 898–906.

16. NCCAM. (2005). *Thinking about complementary and alternative medicine.* National Institutes of Health Publication No. 05–5541.

17. Spross, J. A. (1999). Nondrug intervention for pain management: The magnetic pain drain. *Developments in Supportive Cancer Care, 3*(3), 90–92.

18. Rakel, D., Weil, A. (2007). Philosophy of integrative medicine. In D. Rakel (Ed.), *Integrative medicine* (2nd ed., pp. 5–12). Philadelphia: Saunders.

19. WHO: World Health Organization. (2006, October). *Constitution of the World Health Organization– Basic Documents* (45th ed., Suppl.). Geneva, Switzerland: World Health Organization.

20. Flor, H., Fydrich, T., & Turk, D. C. (1992). Efficacy of multidisciplinary pain treatment centers: A meta-analytic review. *Pain, 49*, 221–230.

21. Karjalainen, K., Malmivaara, A., van Tulder, M., et al. (2003). Multidisciplinary biopsychosocial rehabilitation for subacute low back pain among working age adults. *Cochrane Database Systematic Reviews, 2*, CD002193.

22. Lorig, K. R., Mazonson, P. D., & Holman, H. R. (1993). Evidence suggesting that health education for self management in patients with chronic arthritis has sustained health benefits while reducing health care costs. *Arthritis and Rheumatism, 36*(4), 439–446.

23. Wells-Federman, C. L. (2000). Care of the patient with chronic pain: Part II. *Clinical Excellence for Nurse Practitioners, 4*(1), 4–12.

24. Turk, D. C. (2001). Combining somatic and psychosocial treatment for chronic pain patients: Perhaps 1 + 1 = 3. *Clinical Journal of Pain, 17*:281–283.

25. McCaffery, M., Pasero, C. (1999). *Pain clinical manual* (2nd ed.). St. Louis, MO: Mosby.

26. Kutner, J. S., Smith, M. C., Corbin, L., et al. (2008). Massage therapy versus simple touch to improve pain and mood in patients with advanced cancer: A randomized trial. *Annals of Internal Medicine, 149*(6), 369–379.

27. Cherkin, D. C., Eisenberg, D., Sherman, K. J., et al. (2001). Randomized trial comparing traditional Chinese medical acupuncture, therapeutic massage, and self-care education for chronic low back pain. *Archives of Internal Medicine, 161*(8), 1081–1088.

28. Furlan, A. D., Brosseau, L., Imamura, M., et al. (2002). Massage for low-back pain: A systematic review within the framework of the Cochrane collaboration back review group. *Spine, 27*, 1896–1910.

29. Frey Law, L. A. F., Evans, S., Knudtson, J., et al. (2008). Massage reduces pain perception and hyperalgesia in experimental muscle pain: A randomized, controlled trial. *Journal of Pain, 9*(8), 714–721.

30. Furlan, A. D., Imamura, M., Dryden, T., et al. (2008, October 8). Massage for low-back pain. *Cochrane Database Systematic Review, 4*, No. CD001929.

31. Brosseau, L., Yonge, K. A., Robinson, V., et al. (2003). Thermotherapy for treatment of osteoarthritis. *Cochrane Database of Systematic Reviews, 4*, Art. No. CD004522.

32. French, S., Cameron, M., Walker, B., et al. (2006). Superficial heat or cold for low back pain. *Cochrane Database of Systematic Reviews, 1* Art. No. CD004750.

33. Nadler, S. F., Steiner, D. J., Erasala, G. N., et al. (2002). Continuous low-level heat wrap therapy provides more efficacy than ibuprofen and acetaminophen for acute low back pain. *Spine, 27*(10), 1012–1017.

34. Price, D. D., Riley, J. L., & Wade, J. B. (2001). Psychological approaches to measurement of the dimensions and stages of pain. In D. C. Turk & R. Melzack (Eds.), *Handbook of pain assessment* (2nd ed., pp. 53–75). New York: The Guilford Press.

35. Arnstein, P., Caudill, M., Mandle, C. L., et al. (1999). Self-efficacy as a mediator of the relationship between pain intensity, disability and depression in chronic pain patients. *Pain, 80*(3), 483–491.

36. Evans, S., Weinberg, B. A., Spielman, L., et al. (2003). Assessing negative thoughts in response to pain among people with HIV. *Pain, 105*(1–2), 239–245.

37. Wells-Federman, C. L., Struart-Shor, E., Webster, A. (2001). Cognitive therapy: Applications for health promotion, disease prevention and disease management. *Nursing Clinics of North America, 36*(1), 93–114.

38. Caudill, M. A. (2002). *Managing pain before it manages you* (rev. ed.). New York: Guilford Press.

39. Arnstein, P. M. (2007, June 26). Lessons from Mrs. Tandy: Learning to "live with" chronic pain. *Topics in Advanced Practice Nursing* [ejournal], *7*(1). Retrieved July 2, 2007 from http://www.medscape.com/viewarticle/557719_4

40. Wiech, K., Farias, M., Kahane, G., et al. (2008). An fMRI study measuring analgesia enhanced by religion as a belief system. *Pain, 139*(2), 467–476.

41. Hanson, L. C., Dobbs, D., Usher, B. M., et al. (2008). Providers and types of spiritual care during serious illness. *Journal of Palliative Medicine, 11*(6), 907–914.

42. So, P. S., Jiang, Y., & Qin, Y. (2008). Touch therapies for pain relief in adults. *Cochrane Database Systematic Reviews, 4*, No. CD006535.

43. Giasson, M., & Bouchard, L. (1998). Effect of therapeutic touch on the well-being of persons with terminal cancer. *Journal of Holistic Nursing, 16*(3), 383–398.

44. Gordon, A., Merenstein, J. H., D'Amico, F., Hudgens, D. (1998). The effects of therapeutic touch on patients with osteoarthritis of the knee. *Journal of Family Practice, 47*(4), 271–277.

45. Bossi, L. M., Ott, M. J., & DeCristofaro, S. (2008). Reiki as a clinical intervention in oncology nursing practice. *Clinical Journal of Oncology Nursing, 12*(3), 489–494.

46. Smith, D. W., Arnstein, P. M., Rosa, K. C., et al. (2002). Effects of integrating therapeutic touch into a cognitive behavioral pain treatment program: report of a pilot clinical trial. *Journal of Holistic Nursing, 20*(4), 367–387.

47. Chen, K. W., Perlman, A., Liao, J. G., et al. (2008). Effects of external qigong therapy on osteoarthritis of the knee: A randomized controlled trial. *Clinical Rheumatology, 21*(2), 99–111.

48. Cepeda, M. S., Chapman, C. R., Miranda, N., et al. (2008). Emotional disclosure through patient narrative may improve pain and well-being: Results of a randomized controlled trial in patients with cancer pain. *Journal of Pain and Symptom Management, 35*(6), 623–631.

49. Morone, N. E., Lynch, C. S., Greco, C. M., et al. (2008). "I felt like a new person." The effects of mindfulness meditation on older adults with chronic pain: Qualitative narrative analysis of diary entries. *Journal of Pain, 9*(9), 841–848.

50. Weir, R., & Nielson, W. R. (2001). Interventions for disability management. *Clinical Journal of Pain, 17*(4 Suppl.), S128–S132.

51. Diers, D. (1972). The effect of nursing interaction on patients in pain. *Nursing Research, 21*(5), 419–428.

52. Arnstein, P. M. (2003). The placebo effect. *Seminars in Integrative Medicine, 1*(3), 125–135.

53. Seeley, D. (1990). Selected nonpharmacologic therapies for chronic pain: The therapeutic use of the placebo effect. *Journal of the American Academy of Nurse Practitioners, 2*(1), 10–16.

54. Thomas, K. B. (1987). General practice consultations: Is there any point to being positive? *British Medical Journal, 294,* 1200–1202.

55. Linton, S. J., Hellsing, A. L., & Larsson, I. (1997). Bridging the gap: Support groups do not enhance long-term outcomes in chronic back pain. *Clinical Journal of Pain, 13*(3), 221–228.

56. Subramaniam, V., Stewart, M. W., & Smith, J. F. (1999). The development and impact of a chronic pain support group: A qualitative and quantitative study. *Journal of Pain and Symptom Management, 17*(5), 376–383.

57. Arnstein, P. M., Vidal, M., Wells-Federman, C., et al. (2002). From chronic pain patient to peer: Benefits and risks of volunteering. *Pain Management Nursing, 3*(3), 94–103.

58. Arnstein, P. M., Caudill, M. A., Wells-Federman, C. L. (2000). Self-efficacy as a mediator of depression and pain-related disability in different samples of chronic pain patients. *Progress in Pain Research and Management, 4,* 1105–1111.

Chapter 8: Advanced Techniques and Technologies for Pain Control

1. Weber, R. J. (2007). Developing quality indicators for patient controlled analgesia. In M. R. Cohen, R. J. Weber & J. Moss, *Patient controlled analgesia: Making it safer for patients.* Retrieved December 10, 2008 from http://www.ismp.org/ce/default.asp

2. Joint Commission. (2006, April 3). Tubing misconnections—A persistent and potentially deadly occurrence. *Sentinel Event Alert, 36.* Retrieved December 29, 2008 from http://www.jointcommission.org/SentinelEvents/SentinelEventAlert/sea_36.htm

3. Simmons, B., Phillips, M. S., Grissinger, M., & Becker, S. C. (2008). Error-avoidance recommendations for tubing misconnections when using luer-tip connectors: A statement by USP safe medication use expert committee. *The Joint Commission Journal on Quality and Patient Safety, 34*(5), 293–296.

4. American Pain Society. (2008). *Principles of analgesic use in the treatment of acute pain and cancer pain* (6th ed.). Glenview, IL: APS Press.

5. Fine, P. G., & Portenoy, R. K. (2007). *A clinical guide to opioid analgesia.* New York, NY: Vendome Group, LLC.

6. Weinstein, E., Arnold, R., & Weissman, D. E. (2006). Opioid infusions in the imminently dying patient. *Fast Fact and Concept* (No. 54). Retrieved December 15, 2008 from http://www.eperc.mcw.edu/FastFactPDF/Concept%20054.pdf

7. Viscusi, E. R. (2008). Patient controlled drug delivery for acute postoperative pain management: A review of current and emerging technologies. *Regional Anesthesia and Pain Medicine, 33*(2), 146–158.

8. Hankin, C. S., Schein, J., Clark, J. A., & Panchal, S. (2007). Adverse events involving intravenous patient controlled analgesia. *American Journal of Healthcare System Pharmacists, 64*, 1492–1499.

9. Joint Commission. (2004, December 20). Patient controlled analgesia by proxy. *Sentinel Event Alert, 33.* Retrieved December 29, 2008 from http://www.jointcommission.org/SentinelEvents/SentinelEventAlert/sea_33.htm

10. Wuhrman, E., Cooney, M., Dunwoody, C., et al. (2007). Authorized and unauthorized ("PCA by proxy") dosing of analgesic infusion pumps: Position statement with clinical practice recommendations. *Pain Management Nursing, 8*(1), 4–11.

11. Pasero, C. (2003). *Intravenous patient controlled analgesia for acute pain management: Self-directed learning module.* Lenexa, KS: American Society for Pain Management Nursing.

12. Banks, A. (2007). Innovations in postoperative pain management: Continuous infusion of local anesthetics. *AORN Journal, 85*(5), 904–914.

13. Chu, C. R., Izzo, N. J., Coyle, C. H., et al. (2008). The in vitro effects of bupivacaine on articular chondrocytes. *Journal of Bone & Joint Surgery, 90*(6), 814–820.

14. Pasero, C. (2005). *Epidural analgesia for acute pain management in adults: Self-directed learning module.* Lenexa, KS: American Society for Pain Management Nursing.

15. Perry, A. G., & Potter, P. A. (2006). Epidural analgesia. In *Clinical nursing skills & techniques* (6th ed., pp. 144–151). St. Louis: Elsevier Mosby.

16. Muir, M. R., Sullivan, F. L., Dear, G., & Ginsburg, B. (1997). Monitoring practices following epidural analgesics for pain management: A follow-up survey. *Journal of Pain and Symptom Management, 14*(1), 36–44.

17. Viscusi, E. R. (2005). Emerging techniques in the management of acute pain: Epidural analgesia. *Anesthesia & Analgesia, 101*, S23–S29.

18. Ahmed, S. (2006). Intrathecal drug delivery for chronic pain management. In J. Mao (Ed.), *Translational pain research* (Vol. 1). New York: Nova Science Publishers, Inc.

19. Ahmed, S.(2005). Patient selection and trial methods for intraspinal drug delivery for chronic pain: A national survey. *Neuromodulation, 8*(2), 112–120.

20. Deer, T. (2007). Complications associated with intrathecal drug delivery systems. In J. Neal & J. Rathmell (Eds.), *Complications in regional anesthesia and pain medicine.* Philadelphia: Saunders Elsevier.

21. Holmfred, A., Vikerfors, T., Berggren, L., & Gupta, A. (2006). Intrathecal catheters with subcutaneous port systems in patients with severe cancer-related pain managed out of hospital: The risk of infection. *Journal of Pain and Symptom Management, 31*(6), 568–572.

22. Deer, T., Krames, E. S., Hassenbusch, S. J., et al. (2007). Polyanalgesic consensus conference of 2007: Recommendations for the management of pain by intrathecal (intraspinal) drug delivery: Report of an interdisciplinary expert panel. *Neuromodulation, 10*(4), 300–328.

23. Caraway, D., Saulino, M., Fisher, R., et al. (2008). Intrathecal therapy trials with ziconotide. *Practical Pain Management, 8*(2), 53–56.

24. Scanlon, G. C., Moeller-Bertram, T., Romanowsky, S. M., & Wallace, M. S. (2007). Cervical transforaminal epidural steroid injections: More dangerous than we think? *Spine, 32*(11), 1249–1256.

25. Sehgal, N. V. R., Shah, R., McKenzie-Brown, A., & Everett, C. (2005) Diagnostic utility of facet (zygapophyseal) joint injections in chronic spinal pain: A systematic review of evidence. *Pain Physician, 8*(2), 211–224.

26. Nath, S., Nath, C. A., & Pettersson, K. (2008). Percutaneous lumbar zygapophyseal (facet) joint neurotomy using radiofrequency current, in the management of chronic low back pain: A randomized double-blind trial. *Spine, 33*(12), 1291–1297.

27. Mailis-Gagnon, A., Furlan, A. D., Sandoval, J. A., Taylor, R. (2004). Spinal cord stimulation for chronic pain. *Cochrane Database Systematic Review*, (3), No. CD003783.

28. Kumar, K., Wilson, J. R. (2007). Factors affecting spinal cord stimulation outcome in chronic benign pain with suggestions to improve success rate. *Acta Neurochirugica Supplement, 97*(1), 91–99.

29. Visiongain. (2007). *Global pain pharmaceutical market analysis and forecasts 2007–2022.* Retrieved September 21, 2008 from http://www.visiongain.com/report_license.aspx?rid=232

30. Rice, J. (2008, January 28). Gene therapy for chronic pain: Researchers use gene therapy to stop pain signals before they reach the brain. *Technology Review*, [MIT pub.]. Retrieved September 20, 2008 from http://www.technologyreview.com/Biotech/20118/?a=f

31. Schwarz, F., Aoki, A., Becker, J., et al. (2008). Laser application in non-surgical periodontal therapy: A systematic review. *Journal of Clinical Periodontology, 35* (8 Suppl.), 29–44.

32. Oken, O., Kahraman, Y., Ayhan, F., Canpolat, S., Yorgancioglu, Z. R., & Oken, O. F. (2008). The short-term efficacy of laser, brace, and ultrasound treatment in lateral epicondylitis: A prospective, randomized, controlled trial. *Journal of Hand Therapy, 21*(1), 63–68.

33. Yousefi-Nooraie, R., Schonstein, E., Heidari, K., et al. (2008). Low level laser therapy for nonspecific low-back pain. *Cochrane Database Systematic Review*, 16(2), No. CD005107.

34. Jamtvedt, G., Dahm, K. T., Christie, A. , et al. (2008). Physical therapy interventions for patients with osteoarthritis of the knee: An overview of systematic reviews. *Physical Therapy, 88*(1),123–136.

35. Fregni, F., Freedman, S., & Pascual-Leone, A. (2007). Recent advances in the treatment of chronic pain with non-invasive brain stimulation techniques. *Lancet Neurology, 6*(2), 188–191.

36. MacLachlan, M., McDonald, D., & Waloch, J. (2004). Mirror treatment of lower limb phantom pain: A case study. *Disability and Rehabilitation, 26*(14/15), 901–904.

37. Halligan, P. W., & Berger A. (1999). Phantoms in the brain. *British Medical Journal, 319*, 587–588.

38. Lang, N. M., Hook, M. L., Akre, M. E., et al. (2006). Translating knowledge-based nursing into referential an executable applications in an intelligent clinical information system. In C. A. Weaver, C. W. Delaney, P. Weber, & R. Carr (Eds.), *Nursing and informatics for the 21st century: An international look at practice, trends and the future* (pp. 291–303). Chicago: HIMMS Press.

39. Berman, R. L. H., Iris, M. A., Bode, R., et al. (2009). The effectiveness of online mind-body intervention for older adults with chronic pain. *Journal of Pain, 10*(1), 68–79.

40. Wells-Federman, C., Arnstein, P. M., & Caudill-Slosberg, M. A. (2002). Nurse-led pain-management program: Effect on self-efficacy, pain intensity, pain-related disability and depressive symptoms in chronic pain patients. *Pain Management Nursing, 3*(5), 141–153.

41. Friedman, R., Myers, P., Sobel, D., Caudill, M. A., & Benson, H. (1995). Behavioral medicine, clinical health psychology and cost offset. *Health Psychology, 14*(6), 509–518.

Chapter 9: Controlling Pain in Specific Patient Populations

1. Centers for Disease Control and Prevention. (2007). Inpatient procedures. *Fast Facts A-Z* Retrieved November 7, 2008 from http://www.cdc.gov/nchs/FASTATS/insurg.htm and http://www.cdc.gov/nchs/data/nhsr/nhsr004.pdf

2. Ries, L. A. G., Melbert, D., Krapcho, M., et al. (Eds). (2008) *SEER cancer statistics review, 1975-2005, 39.* Bethesda, MD: National Cancer Institute. Retrieved December 1, 2008 from http://seer.cancer.gov/csr/1975_2005/

3. Martin, B. I., Deyo, R. A., Mirza, S. K., et al. (2008). Expenditures and health status among adults with back and neck problems. *JAMA, 299*(6), 656–664.

4. Centers for Disease Control and Prevention. (2008). Targeting arthritis: Improving quality of life for more than 46 million Americans. *At a Glance 2008.* Retrieved December 1, 2008 from http://www.cdc.gov/nccdphp/publications/aag/arthritis.htm

5. National Center for Health Statistics. Health, United States. (2006). *Special feature on pain with chartbook on trends in the health of Americans.* Hyattsville, MD: Centers for Disease Control and Prevention. Retrieved November 20, 2008 from http://www.cdc.gov/nchs/data/hus/hus06.pdf

6. American Academy of Pediatrics and Canadian Paediatric Society. (2006). Policy statement: Prevention and management of pain in the neonate: An update. *Pediatrics, 118*(5), 2231–2241.

7. Leifer, G. (2008). *Maternity nursing: An introductory text* (10th ed., pp. 144–148). Riverside, CA: Saunders.

8. Amin, S. B., Sinkin, R. A., Glantz, J. C. (2007). Metaanalysis of the effect of antenatal indomethacin on neonatal outcomes. *American Journal of Obstetrics and Gynecology, 197*(5), 486, e1–e10.

9. Anim-Somuah, M., Smyth, R., & Howell, C. (2005, October). Epidural versus non-epidural or no analgesia in labour. *Cochrane Database of Systematic Reviews, 4*, No. CD000331.

10. Leo, S., & Sia, A.T. (2008). Maintaining labour epidural analgesia: What is the best option? *Current Opinion in Anaesthesiology, 21*(3), 263–269.

11. Food and Drug Administration. (2007, August 17). *FDA warning on codeine use by nursing mothers.* Retrieved December 2, 2008 from http://www.fda.gov/bbs/topics/NEWS/2007/NEW01685.html

12. Anand, K. J. S., & Hickey, P. R. (1987). Pain and its effect in the human neonate and fetus. *New England Journal of Medicine, 317*, 1321–1329.

13. Taddio, A., Katz, J., Ilersich, A. L., et al. (1997). Effect of neonatal circumcision on pain response during subsequent routine vaccination. *Lancet, 349*, 599–603.

14. American Academy of Pediatrics. (2000). Prevention and management of pain and stress in the neonate. *Pediatrics, 105*(2), 454–461.

15. Anand, K. J. S. (2008). Analgesia for skin-breaking procedures in newborns and children: What works best? *Canadian Medical Association Journal, 179*(1), 11–12.

16. Taddio, A., Shah, V., Hancock, R., et al. (2008). Effectiveness of sucrose analgesia in newborns undergoing painful medical procedures. *Canadian Medical Association Journal, 179*(1), 37–43.

17. Simons, S. H., van Dijk, M., Anand, K. J. S., et al. (2003). Do we still hurt newborn babies? A prospective study of procedural pain and analgesia in neonates. *Archives of Pediatric & Adolescent Medicine, 157*(11), 1058–1064.

18. American Medical Association. (2007). *Pediatric pain management* [online series] (Module 6). Retrieved December 1, 2008 from http://www.ama-cmeonline.com/pain_mgmt/module06/index.htm

19. Miaskowski, C., Cleary, J., Burney, R., Coyne, P., Finley, R., Foster, R., et al. (2005). *Guideline for the management of cancer pain in adults and children* [APS Clinical Practice Guideline Series] (No. 3). Glenview, IL: American Pain Society.

20. Thomas, J., Karver, S., Cooney, G. A., et al. (2008). Methylnaltrexone for opioid-induced constipation in advanced illness. *New England Journal of Medicine, 358*(22), 2332–2343.

21. Brems, C., Johnson, M. E., Wells, R. S., et al., (2002). Rates and sequelae of the coexistence of substance use and other psychiatric disorders. *International Journal of Circumpolar Health 61*(3), 224–244.

22. Heinemann, A. W., Keen, M., Donohue, R., et al. (1988). Alcohol use by persons with recent spinal cord injury. *Archives of Physical Medicine and Rehabilitation, 69*(8), 619–624.

23. Norman, S. B., Tate, S. R., Anderson, K. G., et al. (2007). Do trauma history and PTSD symptoms influence addiction relapse context? *Drug and Alcohol Dependence, 90*(1), 89–96.

24. Rosenblum, A., Joseph, H., Fong, C., et al. (2003). Prevalence and characteristics of chronic pain among chemically dependent patients in methadone maintenance and residential treatment facilities. *JAMA, 289*(18), 2370–2378.

25. American Society of Addiction Medicine. (2001). *Definitions related to the use of opioids for the treatment of pain: A consensus document from the American Academy of Pain Medicine, the American Pain Society, and the American Society of Addiction Medicine.* Glenview, IL: American Academy of Pain Medicine. Retrieved December 2, 2008 from http://www.painmed.org/pdf/definition.pdf

26. American Society for Pain Management Nursing. (2002). *Pain management in patients with addictive disease: A position paper.* Retrieved December 2, 2008 from http://www.aspmn.org/Organization/documents/addictions_9pt.pdf

27. Baron, M. J., & McDonald, P. W. (2006). Significant pain reduction in chronic pain patients after detoxification from high-dose opioids. *Journal of Opioid Management 2*(5), 277–282.

28. Chang, G., Chen, L., Mao, J. (2007). Opioid tolerance and hyperalgesia. *The Medical Clinics of North America 91*(2):199–211.

29. Wasan, A. D., Correll, D. J., Kissin, I., et al. (2006). Iatrogenic addiction in patients treated for acute or subacute pain: A systematic review. *Journal of Opioid Management, 2*(1), 16–22.

30. Pergolizzi, J., Böger, R. H., Budd, K., et al. (2008). Opioids and the management of chronic severe pain in the elderly: Consensus statement of an international expert panel with focus on the six clinically most often used World Health Organization step III opioids (buprenorphine, fentanyl, hydromorphone, methadone, morphine, oxycodone). *Pain Practice, 8*(4), 287–313.

31. American Pain Foundation. (2008). *A reporter's guide: Covering pain and its management.* Baltimore: APF. Retrieved November 30, 2008 from http://www.painfoundation.org/Publications/ReportersGuide2008.pdf

32. Ballantyne, J. C. (2007). Opioid analgesia: Perspectives on right use and utility. *Pain Physician, 10*(3), 479–491.

33. Chou, R., Fanciullo, G. J., Fine, P. G., et al. (2009). Clinical guidelines for the use of chronic opioid therapy in chronic noncancer pain: American pain society & American academy of pain medicine opioids guidelines panel. *Journal of Pain, 10*(2), 113–146.

34. Wells-Federman, C. L. (2000). Care of the patient with chronic pain: Part II. *Clinical Excellence for Nurse Practitioners, 4*(1), 4–12.

35. Mior, S. (2001). Exercise in the treatment of chronic pain. *Clinical Journal of Pain, 17*(Suppl. 4), S77–S85.

36. Caudill, M., Schnable, R., Zuttermeister, P., et al. (1991). Decreased clinic use by chronic pain patients: Response to behavioral medicine intervention. *Clinical Journal of Pain, 7*, 305–310.

37. Moore, J. E., Von Korff, M., Cherkin, D., et al. (2000). A randomized trial of a cognitive-behavioral program for enhancing back pain self care in a primary care setting. *Pain, 88*, 145–153.

38. Abbot, N. C., Harkness, E. F., Stevinson, C., et al. (2001). Spiritual healing as a therapy of chronic pain: A randomized, clinical trial. *Pain, 91*, 79–89.

39. McCracken, L. M. (1998). Learning to live with the pain: Acceptance of pain predicts adjustment in persons with chronic pain. *Pain, 74*, 21–27.

40. Newshan, G. (1998). Is anybody Listening?: A phenomenological study of pain in the hospitalized person with AIDS. *Journal of the Association of Nurses in AIDS Care, 9*, 57–67.

41. Iwata, K., Tsuboi, Y., Shima, A., et al. (2004). Central neuronal changes after nerve injury: Neuroplastic influences of injury and aging. *Journal of Orofacial Pain, 18*(4), 293–298.

42. Crisp, T., Giles, J. R., Cruce, W. L., et al. (2003). The effects of aging on thermal hyperalgesia and tactile-evoked allodynia using two models of peripheral mononeuropathy in the rat. *Neuroscience Letter, 339*(2), 103–106.

43. Mehta, R. H., Rathore, S. S., Radford, M. J., et al. (2001). Acute myocardial infarction in the elderly: Differences by age. *Journal of the American College of Cardiology, 38*, 736–741.

44. Cooper, G. S., Shlaes, D. M., & Salata, R. A. (1994). Intraabdominal infection: Differences in presentation and outcome between younger patients and the elderly. *Clinical Infectious Diseases, 19*, 146–148.

45. Hilton, D., Iman, N., Burke, G. J., et al. (2001). Absence of abdominal pain in older persons with endoscopic ulcers: A prospective study. *American Journal of Gastroenterology, 96*, 380–384.

46. Tresch, D. D. (1998). Management of the older patient with acute myocardial infarction: Difference in clinical presentations between older and younger patients. *Journal of the American Geriatrics Society, 46*, 1157–1162.

47. Ware, L. J., Epps, C., Herr, K., et al. (2006). Evaluation of the revised faces pain scale, verbal descriptor scale, numeric rating scale, and Iowa pain thermometer in older minority adults. *Pain Management Nursing, 7*, 117–125.

48. Hadjistavropoulos, T., Herr, K., Turk, D. C., et al. (2007). An interdisciplinary expert consensus statement on assessment of pain in older persons. *Clinical Journal of Pain, 23*(1), S1–S43.

49. Strassels, S. A., McNicol, E., & Suleman, R. (2008). Pharmacotherapy of pain in older adults. *Clinics of Geriatric Medicine, 24*(2), 275–298.

50. Fick, D. M., Cooper, J. W., Wade, W. E., et al. (2003). Updating the Beers criteria for potentially inappropriate medication use in older adults. *Archives of Internal Medicine, 163*(22), 2716–2724.

51. Kamal-Bahl, S. J., Stuart, B. C., Beers, M. H. (2006). Propoxyphene use and risk for hip fractures in older adults. *American Journal of Geriatric Pharmacotherapy, 4*(3), 219–226.

52. American Geriatrics Society. AGS Panel on the Pharmacological Management of Persistent Pain in Older Persons. (2009) Pharmacological Management of Persistent Pain in Older Persons. *J Am Geriatr Soc.* 2009 Aug, *57*:1331–1346.

53. Morrison, R. S., Magaziner, J., Gilbert, M., et al. (2003). Relationship between pain and opioid analgesics on the development of delirium following hip fracture. *Journal of Gerontology, 58A*(1), 76–81.

54. American Medical Association. (2007). Assessing and treating pain in older adults. *Pain management online series Module 5.* Retrieved November 17, 2008 from http://www.ama-cmeonline.com/pain_mgmt/module05/index.htm

55. Scudds, R. J., & Scudds, R. A. (2005). Physical therapy approaches to the management of pain in older adults. In S. J. Gibson & D. K. Weiner (Eds.), *Pain in older persons* (pp. 223–237). Seattle: IASP Press.

56. Waters, S., Woodward, J. T., & Keefe, F. (2005). Cognitive-behavioral therapy for pain in older adults. In S. J. Gibson & D. K. Weiner (Eds.), *Pain in older persons* (pp. 239–261). Seattle: IASP Press.

57. Sorkin, B. A., Rudy, T. E., Hanlon, R. B., et al. (1990). Chronic pain in old and young patients: Differences appear less important than similarities. *Journals of Gerontology: Psychological Sciences, 45*, 64–68.

ILLUSTRATION CREDITS

Figure 2–1 is reprinted with permission from Penguin Books Ltd.

Figures 3–1 and 3–3 are adapted from Julius, D., & Basbaum, A. I. (2001). Molecular mechanisms of nociception. *Nature, 413*, 203–210.

Figure 3–4 is adapted from Gottschalk, A., & Smith, D. S. (2001). New concepts in acute pain therapy: Preemptive analgesia. *American Family Physician, 63*, 1979–1984.

Figures 4–1A and B are from Litwack, K. (2009). *Clinical coach for effective perioperative nursing care.* Philadelphia: F. A. Davis.

Figure 4–1C is adapted with permission from Gloth, F. M. III, et al. (2001). The functional pain scale: Reliability, validity and responsiveness in an elderly population. *Journal of the American Medical Directors Association, 2*(3):110–114.

Figure 4–1D is adapted with permission from Feldt, K. S. (2000). The checklist of nonverbal pain indicators (CNPI). *Pain Management Nursing, 1*(1), 13–21.

Figure 4–2 is ©2007 Pain Assessment/Reassessment (MPAR). Used with permission of Massachusetts General Hospital.

Figure 4–3 is adapted with permission from Wilson, D., & Hockenberry, M. J. (2008). *Wong's clinical manual of pediatric nursing* (7th ed.). Elsevier Mosby.

Figure 4–4 is adapted with permission from Manworren, R. C. B., & Hynan, L. S. (2003). Practice applications of research. Clinical validation of FLACC: Preverbal patient pain scale. *Pediatric Nursing, 29*(2), 140–146.

Figure 4–5 is adapted with permission from Hicks, C. L., von Baeyer, C. L., Spafford, P., van Korlaar, I., & Goodenough, B. (2001). The Faces Pain Scale–Revised: Toward a common metric in pediatric pain measurement. *Pain, 93*, 173–183.

Figure 4–6 is adapted with permission from Warden, V., Hurley, A. C., & Volicer, L. (2003). Development and psychometric evaluation of the pain assessment in advanced dementia (PAINAD) scale. *Journal of the American Medical Directors Association, 4*(1), 9–15.

Figure 4–7 is adapted with permission from Gelinas, C., Fillion, L., Puntillo, K., Viens, C., & Fortier, M. (2006). Validation of the critical-care pain observation tool in adult patients. *American Journal of Critical Care, 15*(24), 420–427.

Figure 4–8 is adapted with permission from Arnstein, P. M. (2003). Comprehensive analysis and management of chronic pain. *Nursing Clinics of North America, 38*, 403–417.

Figure 6–1 is reprinted with permission of the World Health Organization. Retrieved from http://www.who.int

Index

Note: Page numbers followed by "b" refer to boxed material; page numbers followed by "f" refer to illustrations; and page numbers followed by "t" refer to tables.